The Learning Brain

The Learning Brain

*Memory and Brain
Development in Children*

Torkel Klingberg, MD, PhD

*Professor of Cognitive Neuroscience
Karolinska Institute
Stockholm Brain Institute
Stockholm, Sweden*

Translated by Neil Betteridge

OXFORD
UNIVERSITY PRESS

OXFORD
UNIVERSITY PRESS

Oxford University Press is a department of the University of Oxford.
It furthers the University's objective of excellence in research, scholarship, and
education by publishing worldwide.

Oxford   New York
Auckland   Cape Town   Dar es Salaam   Hong Kong   Karachi
Kuala Lumpur   Madrid   Melbourne   Mexico City   Nairobi
New Delhi   Shanghai   Taipei   Toronto

With offices in
Argentina   Austria   Brazil   Chile   Czech Republic   France   Greece
Guatemala   Hungary   Italy   Japan   Poland   Portugal   Singapore
South Korea   Switzerland   Thailand   Turkey   Ukraine   Vietnam

Oxford is a registered trademark of Oxford University Press in the UK and
certain other countries.

Published in the United States of America by
Oxford University Press
198 Madison Avenue, New York, NY 10016

Library of Congress Cataloging-in-Publication Data
Klingberg, Torkel, 1967–
[Lärande hjärnan. English]
The learning brain : memory and brain development in children / Torkel Klingberg;
translated by Neil Betteridge.
p. cm.
Includes bibliographical references and index.
ISBN 978–0–19–991710–5 (hardcover)
1. Memory in children.   2. Cognition in children.   3. Child development.
4. Learning.   I. Title.
QP406.K55 2013
612.8'233083—dc23
2012012256

9 8 7 6 5 4 3 2
Printed in the United States of America on acid-free paper

Illustrations used with kind permission from:
IBL Bildbyrå/Science Photo Library 31
NordicPhotos/BSIP 16, 19, 62, 76
Scanpix/SVD/Tomas Oneborg 117
All other Figures and Graphs: Stig Söderlind

CONTENTS

PREFACE

It's a hot June day in Manhattan in 2007. On Seventh Avenue, people are jostling in the heat. But down in the conference room where I'm sitting, the light is subdued and the air conditioning seems set to frosty. I've been invited, as one of several neuroscientists, to lecture at a symposium titled "Cognitive Neuroscience and Education." Speaker after speaker projects images of gray brains with orange patches illustrating which areas are active during different tasks. There are a few minutes to go before I'm due up on stage. It's then that I suddenly get cold feet. Exactly how relevant *is* all this research, my own as well as other people's?

Admittedly, I'd accepted the invitation to deliver a talk on the subject. But I should add that I don't take too much persuading if someone else is going to pay for the flight to New York. Had I been asked to talk on "How Neuroscience Can Bring about World Peace," I'd no doubt still have turned up in Manhattan with my suitcase and my PowerPoint presentation—not that that would mean I'd have any great hopes of my research giving rise to some global Shangri-La, of course. But now, just as I'm about to step up to the podium and attempt to convince the audience with my reasoning, the question sinks ever deeper into my mind.

On the one hand, all learning is about something happening in the brain, so what can be more relevant than brain research? On the other hand, just what can I say to a teacher that will improve her ability to teach her class next week?

If what we have learned from cognitive neuroscience could be put to practical use, it would trigger a pedagogical revolution. But if our knowledge cannot be thus translated, what relevance does the research to which I and thousands of other neuroscientists devote our lives then have? Once a question like this has entered one's mind, it's hard to cast aside—and the result, in my case, is this book.

The conference, as I was later to understand, was part of a surge of interest in the links between neuroscience and education. The subject has been discussed in scientific papers and debate articles, at congresses and conferences the world over. Organizations, research centers, and journals have been created to deal exclusively with this issue. What could have triggered this wave of interest in a new pedagogy is the recent fervor that has made research into the child brain one of the hottest fields in cognitive neuroscience. New methods now enable us to study how the infant brain develops and what occurs there during the learning process, and to identify the problems that cause learning difficulties.

Yet interest in a new science of learning is also driven by necessity. There are many statistics to suggest that levels of knowledge in children have stagnated and in some cases receded. Sweden, the United States, and several European countries are losing ground against Asian nations. International assessments of children's reading and mathematical skills are conducted at regular intervals, and in one such (the 2009 PISA [Program for International Student Assessment] study) Sweden ranked twentieth in math, underperforming all participating Asian countries (South Korea, Japan, China) and even many European ones, such as Slovenia, Denmark, Estonia and Finland. The United States ranked twenty-seventh.

If countries such as the United States and Sweden are unable to compete as knowledge nations, on what will we base our economies? It's not surprising, then, that decision makers have started to seek new solutions, and that their gazes have sometimes turned to neuroscience.

Neuroscience already has a degree of influence on theories of child development and learning. In America, a conference on child development was arranged in 1996 at the White House for a select group of neuroscientists, during which Hilary Clinton (wife of then-President Bill Clinton) made reference to some of the latest results in the field. In Britain, experts have been citing neuroscience studies to advocate earlier learning targets. Here, the main question has been the importance of early stimulation and the receptive phases of cerebral development. The way that politicians have interpreted research findings has engendered a focus on early schooling and learning targets, and it has led to preschools, at which three-year-olds are "stimulated" daily with pedagogical toys and flash cards designed to boost their neurological development. The results are, at best, inconclusive.

One problem is that when politicians, teachers, or the general public apply what they believe to be neuroscientific knowledge, it is often misunderstood. Clinton's initiative was perfectly well intentioned, but many academics are doubtful whether the conclusions drawn were the correct ones. The general public seems as resistant to scientific knowledge as they are willing to spread misconceptions, such as that we only use ten percent of our brains, that men think with their left hemisphere while women think with both, and that creativity resides in the right side of the brain. Worse than these misconceptions is the outright misleading education programs that use scientific terminology but use methods without scientific support, such as Brain Education in the United States and Brain Gym in Britain. In the hundreds of schools that apply Brain Gym methodologies, children learn that they can think better if they stimulate the blood flow to their brains by placing their thumbs under their collarbones and massaging the carotid artery. Luckily for them, no one has told them that the only way to massage the carotid artery under the collarbone is with those sharp scissors that mommy won't let them play with.

My interest in children's learning began with a grant I received for leading a major study into child development. The aim of the project was to explore the relationship between brain maturity, the children's environment, their mnemonic development, and their achievements in the classroom. This we were to do by repeatedly examining children and young people between the ages of six and twenty and monitoring their development during the next four years. We decided to conduct the study in Nynäshamn, a town of approximately 13,000 residents an hour's drive south of Stockholm. In many respects, Nynäshamn is like Sweden in miniature: people have roughly the same level of education and earn roughly as much, and, just like everywhere else in the country, roughly thirteen percent of school leavers fail to meet the national standards set for math.

It's June 2009 and I'm standing at the quayside in Nynäshamn watching sailboats come and go, and cars queueing to embark onto the Gotland ferry. My colleagues and I have just met staff from the school in preparation for the next data-gathering session. Over the coming autumn months, seven psychologists will be travelling between schools with their briefcases full of paper, computers, and small plastic toys for use in memory tests. Each child will undergo hours of individual tests of his or her mathematical and reading skills. Almost a hundred will travel north to Huddinge to have a magnetic resonance scan taken of their brain activity and maturity. Almost all of the 350 children will also have their fingers pricked for a drop of blood to be used in analyses of gene variants potentially significant to the development of memory and learning. Teachers and parents will be inundated with questionnaires—and bribed to answer with cinema tickets—about everything from how their children are getting on at school and their own educational backgrounds, to how many hours their children spend in front of the TV, playing computer games, or practicing a musical instrument.

Would we, data in hand, be able to find any answers to the question of what contributes to the fascinating development of children's cognitive powers and learning skills? What are the key factors behind the fact that not all children bloom but wither along the wayside? Why do some have trouble with concentration and mathematics? How do our brains influence our abilities, and how do our environments influence our brains? The data are still being analyzed, but we are already starting to see some correlations that I will be describing here.

Of all the factors we studied, two were of particular interest and were like spiders in the web: long-term memory and working memory. The long-term memory is the memory system that stores learned facts, rules, names, and experiences. It's the memory that stores what we traditionally associate with learning at school: the accumulation of an encyclopaedia of facts and figures.

Working memory, on the other hand, keeps information up front just when we need it and holds relevant items "in our head" when we're solving a problem.

I've been studying working memory for almost my entire academic life. They say that "for a man with a hammer, every problem is a nail." It can also be true that my research, like this book, places too much emphasis on working memory. In my defense, I'd like to point out that I'm not alone in recognizing the importance of working memory, which is becoming increasingly recognized as a critical function by scientists the world over. Focusing on a specific faculty also makes it possible to delve deeper and illustrate how we can progress from an understanding of individual neurons all the way to what occurs in the classroom; and to see how the lowest level patterns are manifested in the highest level perspective. Bridges must be built between education and cognitive neuroscience. Hopefully this book will be one more structural support on the bridges we are building.

ACKNOWLEDGMENTS

I would like to thank everyone who helped in the writing of this book, especially Tobias Nordqvist, who read several early drafts and who was an invaluable sounding board in its presentation. Thanks to Jenny Toll and Theres Lagerlöf, who helped with the editing, and to Ingvar Lundberg and Mats Myrberg for their comments on the chapter on dyscalculia and dyslexia. Töres Theorell reviewed the chapter on stress and Barbro Johansson the chapter on the effects of the early environment. Thanks also to Stina Söderqvist, who helped me with the figures and literature searches on the effects of exercise, and to Hugo Lagercrantz, Åsa Nilsonne, and Jenny Jägerfeldt for their general comments.

Much of the research described in this book has been financed by a grant from the Knut and Alice Wallenberg Foundation ("Learning and Memory in Children and Young Adults"), the Swedish Riksbank Jubilee Fund, and the Swedish Research Council. The studies were coordinated by Jens Gisselgård, Ylva Samuelsson, and Douglas Sjövall. I am grateful to the Swedish Brain Fund for the help and support they give to child brain research in Sweden, and to the Swedish Foundation for Strategic Research (SSF), which generously funds our research. Finally, a big thanks to all the children, parents, and teachers in Nynäshamn, without whom none of our studies would have been possible.

The Learning Brain

CHAPTER 1

✦

Being Unlucky When You Think

The Importance of Working Memory

Organizing the morning's activities and dropping the kids of at nursery in time is hardly rocket science, but that does-n't mean it's not complicated. One September morning when it's time for me to take my youngest daughter to preschool, and when I think that we're finally ready to cycle off, she descends into the hall fully dressed but without shoes or bag. I ask her to go up to her room to put her socks on and get her backpack. A minute later she comes down with her bag and a scrunchy in her hair—but still barefoot. Another patient instruction from me, and when she returns from her room this time she's actually wearing her socks. We're at last ready to leave—if, that is, we can find her backpack.

Remembering instructions is a skill that employs working memory. But working memory has limited capacity and child-ren have even smaller capacities than adults, which we see in the way they find it harder to remember instructions. The longer the instruction, the more likely it is to be forgotten.

Now I'm not claiming that my children have particularly poor working memories. They don't. Similar episodes can plague me, too—even if I do usually remember to put my socks on in the morning. Take the following incident: I'm just about to round off the day's work when I remember my promise to mail an article to a colleague. All I have to do is open my mail server again. As my inbox automatically fills with new messages, I notice a very interesting letter that demands an immediate response. Pleased with myself that I've managed to reply so promptly, I close the program and shut my laptop. My computer has a little diode in the shape of a crescent moon that flashes when it goes into sleep mode. Once it's done that, it takes at least a minute to wake up again. It's when that lamp starts to flash that I realize that after all that, I've forgotten to mail the article to my colleague. Irritated, I boot up my laptop again, write a mail to my colleague and close the lid again. When the little moon starts to flash a second time, I realize that I've forgotten to attach the article.

Similar situations, which I call "working memory gaps," befall every one of us. One reason for this is that we try to keep too much information in the memory at the same time and in so doing exceed its capacity. In the case of my e-mails, it was hopefully not the elementary task of having to remember a single attachment that pushed by working memory beyond its capacity; however, it might well have been the distraction of other interesting messages and the mental composition of my reply that caused the memory of the attachment to fall away. So distractions and irrelevant information constantly threaten to eradicate the relevant information from our working memories; and if this happens a lot to you, there's a reassuring saying: "No, I'm not stupid... I'm just a little unlucky when I think."[1]

REMEMBERING WHAT TO CONCENTRATE ON

In situations involving forgetting to put on socks or to attach a document, many people would describe themselves as unfocused, which in a sense is correct. Working memory and attention are two closely conjugated functions. British psychologist Alan Baddeley, one of the developers of the working memory model, once said that given a second chance, he'd call it "working attention" instead of "working memory."

There are at least three different kinds of attention: arousal, stimulus-driven attention, and controlled attention. The degree of arousal ranges from somnolence to panicky stress. It affects almost everything we do, and in Chapter 8 I'll be describing how important optimal arousal is to working memory and the effects of stress.

Stimulus-driven attention is that which is involuntarily attracted to something unexpected or particularly interesting in our immediate environment. It might be a sudden sound or a person walking past our open office door, but it could equally be thoughts that pop into our head and that we can't help pursuing.

The third type of attention is controlled attention, which we use when we settled down to concentrate on a specific task. It could be the text in the book in our hands, the speaker at the front of the room or that document that we simply must attach to our e-mail...

Of these three types of attention, it's controlled attention that overlaps with working memory, as we must always remember what we have to concentrate upon. Put another way: we keep the information in working memory by constantly concentrating on it. The point is that, even at a neuronal level, it's impossible to distinguish between the faculties of controlled attention and working memory. This is a theme that I explore more thoroughly in my other book, *The Overflowing Brain*.

WHY DO STUDENTS DAYDREAM?

Why do we often see students daydreaming and gazing out of the window instead of listening to the teacher or concentrating on their work? Have they forgotten what it is they have to concentrate on? In an attempt to find the answer to this question, Michael Kane from the University of North Carolina at Greensboro, examined how students' powers of concentration varied over the course of a day.[2] The students had to carry a little pager around wherever they went, and when it beeped they were to fill in a questionnaire about what they were doing at that very moment. Kane was particularly interested in finding out whether the students were concentrating on the task they were meant to be performing and if this activity was cognitively demanding. He also separately measured their working memory capacity by seeing how much information they could keep in their heads before they started making mistakes.

What Kane discovered was that when a task was mentally demanding and lay claim to a portion of working memory, the students within the lower working memory bracket started to find it hard to concentrate and were increasingly inclined to reply that their mind had been wandering. Daydreaming is no doubt good for us at times. Perhaps letting our thoughts fly and maintaining a balance between mental control and mind wandering can stimulate our creativity. Kane found, however, that people with a higher working memory capacity were better able to maintain their focus even during challenging activities. *They remembered what they had to concentrate on.*

Kane's study, and a number of other studies, demonstrate how closely working memory, attention, and distractibility are related. Working memory is largely synonymous with the ability to control attention, and distractions, such as irrelevant e-mails, constitute one of the greatest threats to our ability to retain relevant information. People with lower storage capacity are also more sensitive to distractions. So it's not hard to imagine that abilities such as keeping relevant information in the head, concentrating, and ignoring distractions should be of significance for a child's aptitude in the classroom. Previous studies have shown that working memory is very useful for solving the type of problems posed in IQ tests; however, for our Nynäshamn study, our hypothesis was that the children's working memory was also important for their performance on tests of reading and mathematical skills, and perhaps for the learning process itself (i.e., for how the individuals improved with time). Another point of inquiry that interested us was possible differences in abilities between boys and girls. There is some evidence of gender differences in certain special tests that require visualizing how objects are manipulated in space (visuospatial ability), whereby, on average, males perform better than females, albeit with a considerable overlap in results. There are also verbal tests on which females, on average, outperform males.

So what about the verbal and visuospatial working memory in children? And if there were differences, were they something that developed gradually? If "women are from Venus and men are from Mars," where do the girls and boys of Nynäshamn come from?

THE WORKING MEMORIES OF THE NYNÄSHAMN CHILDREN

In the pursuit of daily life we make frequent use of working memory to remember what to do next. In the pursuit of research, it's used for more artificial tasks. Such tasks might seem meaningless, but they've proved able to provide vital measures of the amount of relevant information that an individual can retain in his or her memory. In Nynäshamn we used both a verbal and a visual working memory task.

For the verbal task, we read out a series of numbers, such as "8...3...5," which the child was to try to remember and repeat in reverse order: "5...3...8." When a child had managed a certain difficulty level, we increased the number of digits and changed the sequence: "6...2...9...1." The test continued until the child failed the task more than fifty percent of the time at a particular level of difficulty, which gave us a capacity limit for how much information he or she was able to retain in working memory.

The task is simple enough for a six-year-old to understand. A bored ten-year-old boy even felt affronted by the overexplicit instructions. When the psychologist slowly explained the task to him: "And then I'll be saying some numbers, 8-5-2, and I'll want you to repeat them backwards to me. Do you think you can do that?" he replied "owt-evif-thgie" without once pausing in his ceaseless enterprise of spinning on his chair.

For the visual working memory task, we used a computer program that generated a four-by-four grid of sixteen squares into which circles would randomly appear. The children simply had to observe the sequence and repeat it by clicking on the appropriate boxes, a task that became progressively difficult as the sequences increased in length. The information that the children

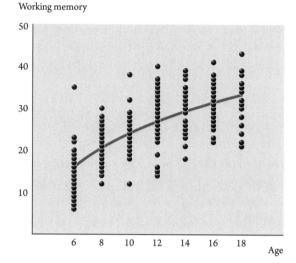

Figure 1.1 Age and working memory (number of correct answers on a visuospatial working memory test) in children and young adults in the Nynäshamn study. Each dot represents an individual.

were to keep in their minds was therefore not just visual but also spatial.

Figure 1.1 shows the results from the first study of working memory. It is a fascinating graph with two clear messages to tell. First, it shows that there is an enormous increase in working memory capacity throughout childhood, all the way into the teens. From the age of six to seven, this capacity grows by twenty percent—a dynamic development of which in later years we can but dream. The second is that there is enormous individual variation. Consider, for instance, the group of ten-year-olds. Some perform at the average level of a fourteen-year old, others at that of a six-year-old. To be sure, all data contains elements of chance and noise, especially data derived from a single experiment. But even when we combine the results from several working memory tests conducted on different occasions, only a little of that variation is erased.

Our next step was to analyze whether the results of our working memory test were related to the children's achievements in math and reading at school.

The strength of a dependency or association is typically expressed in terms of the correlation coefficient, or *r* value. An *r* value of

0 means that there's no relationship between two factors, such as share prices and air humidity. An *r* value of 1, on the other hand, means that two factors are in a state of total dependency.

The correlation between the mathematical skills and visuospatial working memory of the Nynäshamn children turned out to be 0.62, which in psychological contexts is very high. This means that roughly forty percent of the differences in mathematical skills between children is attributable to differences in working memory. But their results on the math test also correlated highly with verbal working memory, reasoning, and reading skills. There was no link, however, to performance on a test of long-term memory involving recalling faces or words.

We now turned our spotlight on predictors of the children's mathematical development. As it turned out, it was the visuospatial working memory that proved the most important factor in this, so a child with relatively high working memory capacity not only performed better at math but also improved at a faster pace.

The next step was to compare the performances of girls and boys on the visuospatial working memory task. No difference! Despite the fact that we had several hundred individuals in the analysis, there wasn't the slightest trend toward gender variation. Nor was there a trend toward a difference for the verbal working memory task. We then compared mathematical performance between the sexes. No difference! So in other words, there were huge variations between how well children achieved, but the sex to which they belonged simply was not an explanatory factor.

We also measured reading comprehension with a series of tests, including one in which the children had to read passages and answer questions. Performance on these tests were also associated to both verbal and visual working memory but not to long-term memory. Reading, of course, requires a long-term memory—so that we can understand what words mean, for one thing. But our results suggest that long-term memory variations in children were not what determined their level of reading comprehension.

The first hypothesis in our theory seemed to be holding: working memory is key to mathematical skills and reading comprehension, and not just for a child's performance on an isolated occasion but for his or her long-term development. The enormous variation in capacity is a crucial factor to keep in mind, not least for teachers seeking contact with a class of children whose working memory capacities might well span a range corresponding to several years' development. So what characterizes children with low working memories and what can we do to help them?

ATTENTION-DEFICIT/HYPERACTIVITY DISORDER AND CHILDREN WITH LOW WORKING MEMORIES

We all know how irritating it is to stumble into a working memory gap. What would life be like if we kept suffering them a hundred times a day? British psychologist Susan Gathercole has studied children whose working memory falls in the lowest ten percentile; here she describes one such case[3]:

> Nathan is in his second year of full-time education. He is a quiet child who is well-behaved in the classroom and is relatively popular with his peers. He has been placed in the lowest ability groups in both reading and math. His teacher feels that he often fails to listen to what she says to him, and says that she often feels that he is "in a world of his own."
>
> In class, Nathan struggles to keep up with many classroom activities. For example, when the teacher wrote on the board "Monday 11th November" and underneath, "The Market," which was the title of the piece of work, he lost his place in the laborious attempt to copy the words down letter by letter, writing *moNemarket*. It seemed that he had begun to write the date, forgot what he was doing and began writing the title instead. He also frequently failed to complete structured learning activities. In one instance, when the teacher handed Nathan his computer login cards and told him to go and work on the computer numbered 13, he failed to do this because he had forgotten the number.

Nathan illustrates, among other things, the trouble some children have following instructions, which was one of the most salient problems Gathercole recorded.[4] Something else the researchers noted was that these children seriously struggled with math and reading, so much so that around eighty percent of them failed to pass the key stage for their year. They were often called "unfocused" by their teachers and typically accused of "not listening to a word I say" or that "it's in one ear and out of the other." Yet not one teacher complained of the children having poor memories.

Since many of the symptoms described by the teachers are associated with attention problems, Gathercole and her colleagues used rating scales to assess symptoms normally associated with attention-deficit/hyperactivity disorder (ADHD). These symptoms fall into two categories, one concerning hyperactivity and impulsive behavior, such as an inability to sit still, while the other shows symptoms of attention difficulties, such as an inability to fix the mind on a task for a longer period of time. Given that working memory and attention are overlapping concepts, it was conceivable that children with low working memories would also display a number of ADHD symptoms. On the whole, children with low working memories did indeed have more such symptoms than other children. However, while as many as seventy-five percent had attention problems identified by the questionnaire, it was only a minority who had serious difficulties with hyperactivity and impulsiveness.

Children diagnosed with ADHD perform on average much more poorly on working memory tests than other children, particularly on the visuospatial tasks. But studies by psychologists like Gathercole show that ADHD and low working memory are far from synonymous, and if we look at individually objectively rated working memory, we can identify another group of children who are not best categorized with the classical ADHD symptoms. Furthermore, the children with low working memories displayed a different gender pattern than that seen with ADHD. Whereas roughly as many boys as girls have a low working memory, the proportion of girls with an ADHD diagnosis is consistently lower, typically around twenty percent. ADHD diagnostics thus overlook many girls with working memory deficits and focus more on hyperactivity—which although often disturbing for parents and teachers and partly treatable with medication, does not necessarily have any bearing on the child's cognitive abilities or predicted educational achievements.

The ADHD diagnosis is thus not synonymous with "children with low working memories." To be better able to identify children with low working memories, Gathercole devised a separate questionnaire called *The Working Memory Rating Scale* to measure their ability to remember an instruction and to carry out a sequence of tasks, and thus to isolate and pin down the specific behavior traits that she observed in them. For instance, there were questions asking whether the child "abandons an activity before it reaches completion," "often loses his/her place in longer activities that require multiple steps," "finds it hard to concentrate" or "shows poor linguistic and mathematical development."

Other categories of question that revealed particular discrepancies between children concerned initiation (i.e., the ability to initiate an activity). Could it be that this is linked to problems formulating a plan for a particular behavior and then retaining this plan in working memory?

Gathercole's study also showed that children with low working memories also had poorer self-esteem, having self-rated themselves lowest in terms of "personal power," which is shorthand for the perception a person has of his or her ability to influence his or her immediate surroundings. Not so surprising, perhaps, for individuals who are constantly suffering gaps in their working memory and struggling with core subjects in the classroom. But low self-esteem can set off a negative spiral. So having your problems explained can be of intrinsic value in and of itself, just like for other problems such as ADHD, as the title of a self-help book perfectly encapsulates: *You mean I'm not lazy, stupid, or crazy?*[5]

It is particularly important to identify children with low working memories if doing so can incite practical measures. Rosemary Tannock, cognitive neuroscientist at the University of Toronto, has been a driving force in the development of a pedagogical method specifically for children with working memory deficits. Her method involves educating teachers about the nature of working memory, what aspects of schoolwork demand working memory capacity, and the consequences that can be expected of working memory deficits.[6]

The education also provides a range of strategies designed to make it easier for children to learn despite a poor working memory. In most cases, the method entails reducing the demands on working memory and supplying external aids to relieve them of some of the information burden. For example, the children might be given briefer instructions that don't overload their capacity (reducing demands) and notes or pictures that remind them of a sequence of actions so that they don't have to keep the information active in their working memories (external aids). Another crucial expedient is to reduce the number of distractions, which can be done by fitting the children with earphones or their desks with screens. The strain on working memory is thus minimized, which is the key point of this educational theory. There is another interesting approach, namely to augment working memory through training, and this is something that I'll be discussing in Chapter 9.

The initial results of the Nynäshamn study confirmed the importance of working memory, but they also raise several questions. What causes the enormous spread in capacity among individuals? Which environmental and biological factors impinge upon working memory, and why do we see this strong link between working memory and math?

Unfortunately, my working memory gaps are not growing fewer with the years—far from it. My children, on the other hand, are older and not only do they remember to put on their socks in the morning, they will also soon be able to recall as long a series of instruction as I can. This is good news—for them—but what is it that underlies their, and other children's, working memory development and what might cause it to become impaired?

CHAPTER 2

✧

The Growing Brain

How the Brain Develops and Matures

Laura lives with her parents in the outskirts of Durham, North Carolina.* She's a happy, upbeat, and popular girl, who does well at school and is at the top of her class in both mathematics and reading. But in the autumn of her eighth year everything changes. Laura starts getting ever more frequent headaches, particularly in the morning, and attacks of nausea and vomiting. Her anxious parents take her to the family doctor, who refers her to a neurologist and a magnetic resonance (MR) scan confirms her parents' greatest fear: a brain tumor.

The MR images show that the tumor is located next to the midbrain and is probably a medullablastoma, a malignant tumor especially common in children. The expanding tumor is increasing the pressure inside her skull, and it's this pressure that's creating both the headaches and the nausea. Fortunately, the particular type of tumor has a good prognosis. Surgeons remove it and Laura is given cytostatics and radiotherapy to kill any remaining tumor cells. There is every sign that the operation is a success and that the tumor will not be returning. She is cured.

---

* Laura is not her real name.

The problem, as it turns out, is not so much the tumor as the treatment. Tumors and cancers are caused by uncontrolled cell division, and it's their ability to prevent this process that gives cytostatics and radiation their efficacy. If the same treatment had been given to an adult, the side effects would not have been as serious, but in an eight-year-old's developing body it attacks the natural growth process, too, including that of the brain itself. Just a year after treatment, Laura's school performance deteriorates. Her parents suspect that it is the effect of the stress that the disease and the operation have caused her. But two years afterward, the problems are more pronounced and Laura is finding it hard to organize her schoolwork, so that now—as her mother reports to her doctor—it's taking Laura almost twice as long as her classmates to complete her homework. Four years afterward, the young girl, who was once at the top of the class, has such severe problems that she requires a personal tutor to keep up.

At the hospital, neuropsychologists have been monitoring Laura's cognitive capacity with annual tests of intelligence and working memory. When her scores on these tests are matched with the expected performance of her peers, the most pronounced problems can be suggested for an aggregated score of a working memory test and a mathematics test. Prior to the operation, Laura was way above average, but four years afterward she is far below the expected value. It is not that her working memory is any worse: she has roughly the same working memory capacity. But all her friends are improving at a rate of about ten percent a year, while Laura seems to have halted in her development and is therefore finding it harder and harder to keep up.

No news is good news. Sometimes we only notice a phenomenon when something goes wrong. Laura's case illustrates how important the development of the child brain is. Let us take a closer look at cerebral development and how it might help us understand Laura's problem, and the normal development of children's cognitive functions.

THE DEVELOPMENT OF THE BRAIN

The first signs of a rudimentary brain begin to appear when the fetus is only two weeks old and just a few millimeters long.[1] A small tube grows from a plate of primitive nerve cells that is no more complex than it is during the same development stage of a worm. But the fact of its becoming a tube is a vital process; if it is not closed properly, the spine can rupture and the child can, at worst, be born with part of the spinal cord protruding into a sac on the child's back.

The brain and the spinal cord will form from this tube. The upper part of the tube starts to expand like a balloon into the vesicle that will eventually become the cerebrum. In the middle of the cerebrum is a layer of stem cells that now divide to form new nerve cells, or neurons. These new neurons climb out toward the periphery to form a layer of nerve cell bodies, or soma, on the outside of the cerebrum, which becomes the cortex. The cell division takes place during the tenth to twentieth week and is a particularly sensitive process. Fetuses in this stage of development when the bomb fell on Hiroshima received serious brain injuries, while those a little younger or older fared better.

At first, the cortex is completely smooth, but as more cells are added, it folds in on itself so that it can fit inside the skull.

Attached to the soma are long protrusions called dendrites, like the branches of a tree, which allow neurons to communicate with each other. The point of contact between two neurons is called a synapse, and a single neuron can receive signals from 10,000 such synapses. The different signal potentials are then weighed up by the neuron. In contrast to the complex information that the cell receives from thousands of others, its response is rather limited: it's either passive or transmits a signal. The signal is an electric impulse that's conducted down a thread-like projection called an axon, at the end of which are the synapses that transmit it on to the next neuron. Neurons thus have an extremely limited repertoire of responses—it's in the network that the complexity, information processing, and memory reside.

At birth, most neurons are already in place in the cortex. Then the projections grow and branch, not unlike how the branches of a tree lengthen and fork with age. The complex branching enables new links and networks to be formed. This continues for several years; exactly how long depends on the part of the brain. Technically, it's difficult to obtain an exact measurement, but the branching process probably occurs up to the age of two in some brain areas, and as late as twelve in others (see Fig. 2.1).

During this dynamic growth phase, the brain demands vast amounts of energy. Even the adult brain takes roughly twenty-five percent of the body's energy despite it accounting for only two percent of body weight. In a four-year-old child, the energy consumption of the brain is fifty percent higher than in an adult and the brain also makes up a larger portion of the total body weight.[2]

Following the growth of the protrusions, the number of branches and synapses declines. If we extend the metaphor of the

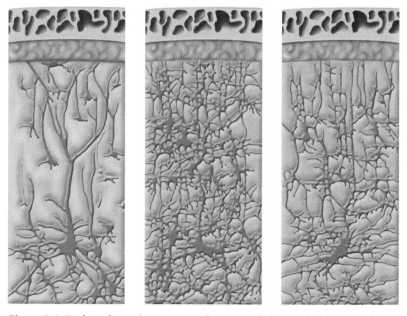

Figure 2.1 The branching of neurons is at first sparse (left), but then becomes denser in early infancy (middle), only to thin out again in later childhood and adolescence (right).

tree, this process is like pruning—which is the very term that scientists use. What probably happens is that a surplus of links is formed and those that are used and contribute to functional networks remain and grow stronger, while those that lack function or are unused are removed.

THE BRAIN MATURES

The volume of the cortex largely consists of these connections and protrusions from the nerve cells, which means that the waxing and waning of branches make the cortex first expand in volume and then shrink. Using detailed anatomical images from a magnetic resonance scanner, scientists can follow these changes in the cortex. If we plot the thickness of the cortex through childhood, we obtain a curve like the one in Figure 2.2. The arrow shows where the cortex is at its thickest. This does not mean it's reached full maturity, but the peak thickness can still provide a kind of indicator of development.

Measurements of the thickness of the cortex and how it changes have proved one of the most important tools in the understanding of brain development during childhood. The key issues are how the degree of maturity of the various parts of the cortex differs with time, how the brain's development relates to cognitive development, what genetic and environmental factors influence the maturing process, and whether developmental aberrations can be the key to understanding behavioral variations.

Figure 2.2 shows the results of a study of children carried out by the National Institute of Mental Health led by Jay Giedd and Philip Shaw, and it illustrates the gradual maturity of the cortex.[3] Here, they use the age of peak thickness to show variations between different parts of the brain. The darker areas show when a certain area has reached its peak thickness and begins to decline. What's interesting is the considerable difference between brain areas; those that reach their peak thickness first are the motor cortex (which controls muscles), the sensory cortex, and the visual cortex at the back. The area that matures last of all is the frontal lobe, or prefrontal cortex.

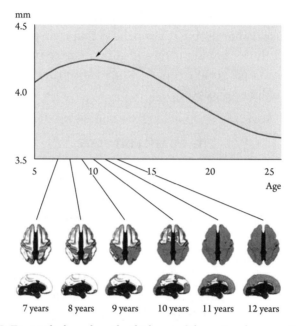

Figure 2.2 The graph shows how the thickness of the cortex changes with the dendritic branching and pruning that occurs during childhood. The arrow indicates the peak thickness, which is a measure of degree of maturity. The brain maps below show how the different parts of the brain mature at different rates (after Shaw et al., 2008). The darker sections show when an area of the brain reaches its peak thickness. The upper row depicts the brain as seen from above (left hemisphere on the left).

So when does the brain reach maturity? When is a child able to manage its child benefit itself or take other important decisions? If we were to use cortical thickness as a gauge of maturity, then "full maturity" would show up as a flattening of the curve in Figure 2.2 into a horizontal line. As we can see in this graph, there is no horizontal part to the curve, at least not before the age of twenty-five. So there is no clear answer to the question of when a certain part of the brain is fully mature; all we see is gradual change and relative differences between cortical areas and individuals.

Cortical thickness can evince several clear gender differences in maturity. Neuroscientists have found that the prefrontal cortex reaches peak maturity at the age of eleven for girls, but twelve for boys (Fig. 2.3 shows where the different lobes are located).[4] For the parietal lobe, the corresponding ages are ten for girls and twelve for boys. Earlier maturity of the frontal lobe in girls seems

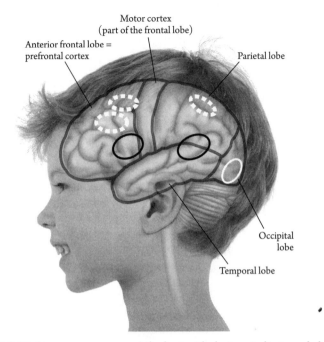

Figure 2.3 Working memory areas of the brain. Black rings indicate verbal areas only; white rings indicate visual areas only; white dotted rings indicate areas that are activated during both verbal and visuospatial working memory tasks.

to tally with the general opinion that girls "mature earlier," but exactly how these differences affect behavior remains unclear. There is also another pattern in the temporal lobe; here, according to the same study,[4] peak thickness is reached at sixteen and a half in boys and seventeen in girls.

When Laura receives her radiotherapy and cytostatics, she's eight years old. The neurons in her frontal lobe should have continued branching for another three years at least at this age, and a disruption of this process could well have been one of the causes of her working memory failure.

So which brain area governs working memory? As there are hundreds of studies of brain activity during working memory tasks, a detailed summary would be difficult to provide. A simplified summary is shown in Figure 2.3.

Visuospatial working memory tests activate visual areas of the occipital lobe. Verbal or sound-based tests of working memory activate the temporal lobe and lower sections of the prefrontal cortex, which are also used for speech. There is also a network of areas in both the parietal and frontal lobes that is activated on verbal and visuospatial working memory tests. In our Nynäshamn study, performances on such tasks were strongly correlated: a child who performed well on the one test did so on the other, too—a parity that would be explained by the presence of common areas for different types of working memory. All working memory tests activate the frontal lobe, and the later maturity of this lobe is arguably one of the most important explanatory factors in the development of working memory during childhood.

There is as yet no study of the maturity of the cortex in children with a low working memory. However, Giedd's team, who had mapped the normal development of the cortex, had also mapped brain development in children with attention-deficit/hyperactivity disorder (ADHD), a group that at least in part overlaps with the group of children with impaired working memories.

When children with and without ADHD were compared, the team noticed large differences in patterns of cerebral development, in that the children with the diagnosis of ADHD showed an almost wholesale delay in brain maturation. The effect was most pronounced in the frontal lobe, with as much as three to seven years' difference between the ages of peak cortical thickness.[5] Part of the phenomenon can thus be attributed to delayed development. Unfortunately, it doesn't seem as if children with ADHD ever catch up. An earlier study, led by Xavier Castellanos, demonstrated that for most areas of the brain, an abnormality remains fixed for life,[6] which means that many of the problems related to attention and working memory endure into adulthood.

GENES AND THE BRAIN

How the growing brain functions and develops determines differences in working memory capacity and other faculties. But this begs the question of why children's brains differ from each other and follow such different maturation trajectories. By studying twins, researchers have found that working memory capacity is largely—at least fifty percent—hereditary.[7],[8] However, it remains unclear exactly which genes are involved. One of the few genes identified as important for working memory (*COMT*) codes for an enzyme that breaks down the neurotransmitter dopamine. Some people have a variant that gives a more rapid degradation, others a variant that gives a slower degradation, yet others a mix of the two, where one gene comes from the mother and one from the father. Slow degradation gives rise to more free dopamine and thus to a better working memory.

In the Nynäshamn study, we studied some fifty genes that had previously been associated with either memory or ADHD. Working alongside Juha Kere's team at Karolinska Institutet in Stockholm, we then examined whether some of the genes had any impact on working memory. What we found was that the gene that codes for the rapid or slow metabolism of dopamine also had an effect in childhood, but one that changed with age.[9] The most likely reason for this is that children have more dopamine than adults and that too much of the neurotransmitter is not good. The "slow-degradation" gene variant was therefore unwelcome in younger children but gave a better working memory around puberty when the dopamine levels had started to drop. This shows how the growing child's brain can obey other "laws" than the adult's. A similar effect has been suggested for the Apo-E gene, of which a particular variant is associated with an increased risk of dementia in elderly people. In young people, however, the same variant seems to have a positive impact on long-term memory.[10],[11]

We also found another gene, *SNAP25*, that had a profound effect on working memory.[12] This gene codes for a protein that is required for a signal to be transmitted between neurons. What was especially interesting about the gene was that it had previously been linked to ADHD. Perhaps this link was really to working memory, problems with which have been misinterpreted as symptomatic of the condition. The results also show that variations within these genes must not be seen as aberrations associated with specific diagnoses in a handful of individuals but as a normal genetic phenomenon that affects large groups of people.

Many might find it provocative to hear about the impact of genes on behavior, and even more so, perhaps, to hear that genes have direct effects on the brain. They will just have to live with it. Genes play a big part in our behavior and our abilities, and they exercise this role via the brain. Our knowledge of genetics is increasing exponentially, and what we're seeing now is just the beginning. But acknowledging the influence of genes is not to deny that of the environment or to claim that the brain is somehow fixed, and I'll be giving many examples of this throughout this book.

THE WHITE MATTER

The description of how the cortex changes over time is but a part of the history of brain maturation. Another, and arguably no less important process, is the development of the white matter. The white matter is a layer of fat (myelin) that sheathes the axons, not unlike insulation encasing electrical wires, and that allows the signal being conducted down the axon to travel faster and more efficiently. Faster conductivity not only creates quicker reaction times but also increases the speed of all information processing. Unlike the complicated developmental pattern of the cortical gray matter, that of the white matter is more straightforward: it constantly increases, and the more myelin the better; and although the steepest part of the growth curve appears around the age of two, the process continues, just like it does for gray matter, all the way into the mid-twenties.

Myelination has been directly linked to the development of cognitive function. In a study that my team and I conducted at Karolinska Institutet, we used a special magnetic resonance technique that can track how the myelin sheath thickens with time. After having examined their white matter, we asked the subjects of the study, who were between seven and eighteen years old, to take tests of working memory and reading comprehension. Doing this, we were able to see that improvements in working memory during childhood correlated with the myelination of several pathway systems in the brain, including those that connect the parietal and frontal lobes (Fig. 2.3).[13],[14] The degree of myelination can vary for several reasons, and according to one study, individuals with a low working memory have thinner myelin sheaths along the axons running between these two lobes.[15]

Different parts of the white matter have different functions and lead different types of information depending on the brain areas they connect. In our study, we found that reading comprehension, measured as the speed at which the subjects could read a list of words, correlated with the maturity of the pathway system that links the anterior and posterior language areas. Interestingly, this is the very same area where we had previously revealed an association between white matter impairment and dyslexia.[16] Knowledge of normal development can thus help us understand the mechanisms behind aberrations and functional impairments.

It's likely that Laura's problem was caused by damage to both her gray and white matter: the nerve branches and connections, and the myelination that ought to have occurred. Significantly, studies of groups of children subjected to similar treatment have revealed lower degrees of white matter myelination. Unfortunately, Laura's prospects are not that hopeful. When researchers in the United States followed up children who had undergone treatment for cancer to see how they were coping as adults, the statistics they produced were depressing.[17] While eighty percent of the control group of young adult Americans had a job and ninety percent a driving licence, less than thirty percent of the cancer-treated group had a job, thirty percent a driving licence, and half as many had their own place to live or were in a relationship.

I heard Laura's story from Kristina Hardy, a neuropsychologist now at the Children's National Medical Center in Washington, DC. She was the first person to examine Laura and monitor her progress. Even though her job is about saving the lives of children with brain tumors, she is also disheartened by the side effects of the treatment and the bearing it has on brain maturity. The problem is that doctors have no idea what to do about the impaired cognitive ability. One way to help these children could be to train their working memory. The outcome of my meeting with Kristina was a project that she set up to see whether training can offset some of the damage caused to the brain. In Chapter 9 I will discuss her findings and show that there might be hope for children in Laura's situation after all.

CHAPTER 3

☙

Through the Pyrenees by Motorbike

The Risk-Taking Teenage Brain

One of the most surprising results of recent research into brain development is how long it carries on. In the 1990s, the National Institute of Mental Health (NIMH) launched a large-scale study on child development that involved monitoring children with regular magnetic resonance scans up to the age of sixteen, the age at which the brain was presumed to be fully developed. To be on the safe side, however, the length of the study was extended to the age of eighteen. Even so, it turned out that they had still missed the end point of brain development by about seven years. Car rental firms, with their detailed databases of accident statistics, often refuse to rent vehicles to anyone under twenty-five, which corresponds with the knowledge we now have of when the brain reaches full maturity. Jay Giedd of the NIMH, one of the most prominent researchers working on the development of the pediatric brain, likes to joke that Hertz obviously has the very best neuroscientists.

The sixteen-year-old brain is not just a less experienced adult brain but an organ that is still under development. Such findings about late cerebral development have sparked interest in the teenage brain. Is it a lack of maturity that explains why a sixteen-year-old decides to test the ski jump on her new BMX? Or why young people are heavily overrepresented in traffic accidents, particularly those involving alcohol or other drugs? I remember how as a young man, I went on a motorbiking holiday with some friends, and we zoomed along narrow mountain roads in the Pyrenees at breakneck speed without helmets. What were we thinking? The motorcycle cops whom we met on the way tapped their fingers meaningfully against their helmets. We assumed that, with their indulgent smiles, they were just telling us to put our helmets on. But perhaps they were also implying that it wasn't only a helmet that was lacking up top but perhaps some common sense and a little white matter, too.

RISKS AND REWARDS

The question occupying the minds of many scientists is whether teenagers assess risks and rewards differently when making decisions. The decision-making process is determined by the reward system and prefrontal cortex, which is able to evaluate signals, make plans, and make decisions. One theory, of which B. J. Casey of the Sackler Institute in New York is a leading proponent, is that these systems mature out of step with each other, the reward system earlier than the prefrontal cortex.[1] This means that teenagers could have a relatively mature reward system but a relatively immature frontal lobe, and therefore act differently to both children (in whom neither of the systems are mature) and adults (in whom both systems are hopefully mature).

Several studies provide evidence that the brain's reward system actually operates differently in teenagers. In one study, a task was used that mimicked playing on a slot machine.[2] Three pictures of fruit would be presented consecutively, perhaps "cherry, kiwi, pear." Three of a kind would mean a win that the participants would receive after the experiment. When two fruits of the same kind had been presented and the participants saw that they had a chance of winning, the reward systems of fourteen- and fifteen-year-olds responded much more actively than those of both younger and older subjects.

In another study, subjects had to choose between two different symbols without knowing in advance the rules that applied and which choices would lead to a lesser or greater reward.[3] Sometimes they were able to predict with a degree of probability that they'd receive a large reward, while at other times rewards were issued randomly and thus would come as a surprise. It was precisely at these times, when the participants received an unexpected payout, that clear variations were manifested between teenagers (ages thirteen to nineteen), children (ages eight to twelve), and adults (ages twenty-five to thirty). The difference in brain activity was localized to a part of the brain called the ventral striatum, an area that receives signals from dopamine-secreting neurons, especially when a reward is anticipated or an unexpectedly large reward is received. The same system is involved in the "reward kick" that drug addiction gives. The investigators' interpretation was therefore that teenagers can be said to be addicted to reward kicks, which might explain why they seek out situations that offer potential rewards despite the risks involved (like riding without a helmet).

The results from behavioral studies of teenagers square with those from brain activation analyses. One major study included over nine hundred people between the ages of seven and thirty.[4] The researchers employed a decision-making test called the *Iowa Gambling Task*, which had previously been used by neurologist Antonio Damasio to show how lesions in the frontal lobe lead to an inability to evaluate risks and rewards. In this test, the subjects are asked to choose cards from four equal decks. Certain cards add or subtract various sums to or from their pot of money. On average, two of the four decks lead to net increases, and gradually the subjects learn to choose cards from the right decks by observing the patterns of wins and losses. As the game progresses, researchers can analyze how the wins and losses gradually change the subjects' gambling behavior.

What they found was the adults were best at adapting their behavior to losses, teenagers next best, and children the poorest. The ability to draw inferences from negative feedback thus develops with age. Gains, on the other hand, influenced the teenagers' choices much more than they did those of the children and adults. Teenagers can plan and assess risks better than children, but the potential rewards exercise an uncontrollably powerful attraction. So the teenage period is not simply a stretch on the path of life between childhood and adulthood, but more of a branch on which cerebral development takes a little detour off the beaten track.

The shift in balance between the prefrontal cortex and the reward system probably exists between the prefrontal cortex and other deeper lying parts of the brain. One such is the amygdala, a collection of nerve cells that plays a key role in fear, anger, and stress. The amygdala is activated when we see images of snakes or read facial expressions depicting anger or hostility, and it is also involved in our own expressions of aggression and fear. Like the reward system, the amygdala is hooked into several other areas of the brain, including the prefrontal cortex, such that activity in the amygdala is integrated with other information in the prefrontal cortex when we take a decision, and activity in the prefrontal cortex can inhibit activity in the amygdala.

William Killgore and Deborah-Yurgelun Todd of Harvard Medical School have advanced the theory that the teenage brain is more driven by emotions than it is by prefrontal control.[5] We know that the amygdala can be involved in exaggerated emotional reactions such as a fear of snakes or sociophobia; might the teenage amygdala be one reason for the intense social sensitivity of the teenage years?

Perhaps we can understand the different reactions of the teenage period from an evolutionary perspective, whereby reckless but rewarding behavior was a necessary part of human development. One advocate of this idea is vet-cum-author David Bainbridge, who proposed it in his book *Teenagers—A Natural History*[6]; and as a vet, it comes naturally to Bainbridge to draw parallels between the teenage periods of humans and other animals. In animals, adolescence is the period during which the individual is to depart its family, even perhaps its social group, to seek new hunting grounds and find a mate. In breaking so completely with a former life, they must take risks and are perhaps disproportionately driven by potential gains. The problem, argues Bainbridge, is that evolutionarily speaking we are prepared for correctly assessing risks involved in climbing tall trees, but not as regards taking crack, sexually transmitted diseases, or the combination of alcohol and wet tarmac.

Jane Goodall, a pioneering observer of chimpanzee behavior, describes how young pubescent males leave their troop to prowl around in gangs terrorizing rivals, with a rather nebulous plan for the future and driven by an instinct that they somehow have to find a mate. A quite fitting description, I feel, of a gang of youths on motorbikes hurtling through the Pyrenees on a vague quest for reward kicks.

NEUROSCIENCE AND THE LAW

There is still far too little research being done about the teenage brain, but it's nonetheless worth pondering over the conclusions we might draw. In some cases, our knowledge of its late development corresponds well with the various policies that exist for young people, such as Hertz's restrictions on car rentals. Should we raise the minimum driving age to twenty-five for everyone? Personally, I really don't think we should. Risks must be weighed up against personal freedom, and it's not always optimal safety that we aspire to. The role that exploratory teenage behavior played 40,000 years ago might still be very relevant, and an accident might well be the price we have to pay for allowing our eighteen-year-old daughter to take the car to the next village to meet her boyfriend. (Although as a parent I'd possibly consider installing an alcohol lock into the car before handing over the keys.)

Car rental firms, who see everyone under the age of twenty-five as immature, are arguably an extreme example of how to appraise the degree of maturity of the young. Another might be laws that treat sixteen-year-olds as inexperienced but otherwise complete versions of adults. In some US states people under the age of eighteen can be sentenced to life imprisonment without parole for non-homicide offences. There are over a hundred such cases of young people serving life sentences around the world, seventy-seven of which are in Florida. The particularly high number in this state is the result of legislation introduced in the 1990s, when politicians observed with alarm a rise in youth crime that risked threatening the tourist industry. In the autumn of 2009 two of these cases were appealed to the Supreme Court on the grounds that the lifetime incarceration of young offenders contravened the constitution's prohibition of "cruel and unusual punishment."

One of the cases concerned a young man called Terrance Graham, who at the age of sixteen robbed a restaurant in Jacksonville and struck the owner with a steel pipe. He was sentenced to a year in prison and three years of probation. During his probationary term, he committed a break-in and was sentenced to life without parole.

His writ to the Supreme Court (*Terrance Jamar Graham v. State of Florida*) cited, among other documents, a statement signed by a dozen international neuroscientists, of which I was one, testifying that there was scientific evidence that at sixteen years old, the human brain is still in a state of development. The scientific argument was summed up as follows:

> ... scientific evidence now sheds light on how and why adolescent behavior differs from adult behavior. The differences in behavior have been documented by scientists along several dimensions. Scientists have found that adolescents as a group, even at later stages of adolescence, are more likely than adults to engage in risky, impulsive, and sensation-seeking behavior. This is, in part, because they overvalue short-term benefits and rewards, are less capable of controlling their impulses, and are more easily distracted from their goals. Adolescents are also more emotionally volatile and susceptible to stress and peer influences. In short, the average adolescent cannot be expected to act with the same control or foresight as a mature adult.

There is much to be said about the influence that neuroscience can or should have on legislation. At one extreme, we could explain most behaviors with reference to brain function. Does this mean that we are no longer accountable, even punishable, for our actions because "it was my brain that did it"? On the other hand, we already allow medical pundits, be they neurologists or psychiatrists, to declare whether someone who has committed a crime was "in full control of his mental faculties" at the time. This is an old and very thorny problem. What's new is that our understanding of the significance of the brain and genes is growing exponentially. Science doesn't only have something to say on extreme cases, such as when injuries produce obvious diseases, but can also pronounce on how normal variation in a person's genetic makeup and brain function shapes the normal variation in his or her behavior and abilities. It might be wise at this very juncture to start discussing what we are to do with this knowledge.

I don't know how impressed the Supreme Court was by our scientific contribution, but it overturned the old law and prohibited the

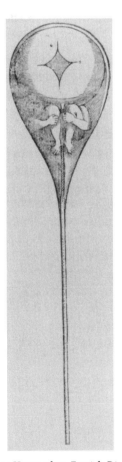

Figure 3.1 Sperm cell. Niklaas Hartsoeker, *Essai de Dioptrique* (1694).

state of Florida from sentencing adolescents to life imprisonment without parole.

A late seventeeth-century scientific illustration depicts a sperm cell containing a tiny miniature baby, hunched up in a fetal position (see Fig. 3.1). The hypothesis, simple and intuitive but entirely wrong, was that babies exist in perfect form from the very beginning and then just increase in size during pregnancy. We now know that the embryonic phase consists of a number of different stages and forms. The fetus begins life as a cluster of cells and then continues through a series of strange metamorphoses, some of which more resemble a tadpole or other evolutionary predecessor than they do a human being.

Similarly, the child's brain is not a complete version of the adult brain that just has to be blown up to the right size. Instead, it's something that's sculpted during at least two decades of growth and cultivation. Children and adolescents must be treated as individuals in a special phase of development, and not as small adults.

This prolonged development also provides a generous window of opportunity for the influences of nurture. "Tend your garden" is a motto that doesn't just encourage us to do a spot of weeding; it also, by analogy, tells us to nurture our interests. Our knowledge of the growth and cultivation of the brain adds yet a third dimension to the expression.

CHAPTER 4

✣

Now I Am Really Awake for the First Time Ever

Long-Term Memory

Clive Wearing contracted a viral infection of the brain at the age of forty-seven, and now, twenty-three years later, has one of the most serious memory impairments ever recorded. He has no memory of the events of the previous day and no memories of his past. Clive doesn't remember that he has adult children, and it takes no more than a few seconds for him to forget what someone has just told him. He keeps a daily diary, in which his entries almost invariably begin with exclamations like: "*Now I am really awake (first time).*"

If working memory connects the thoughts of the moment with the actions of the next, the long-term memory ties together our days and our lives. We use working memory to keep a sequence of instructions in our head, while we use the long-term memory to remember where we live. The long-term memory stores not only factual data on how the world is made up and all the knowledge we painstakingly acquire through study but also the personal experiences that define us as individuals.

A deficient long-term memory presents obvious obstacles to schooling, but it also impacts our daily lives. Take Jon, for example, a thirty-year old man living in a suburb of London. Jon's problem was probably caused by complications stemming from his extremely premature birth in the twenty-sixth week. When he was born, he was blue and apparently lifeless, and tests confirmed abnormally low levels of oxygen, which later proved to cause irreparable damage to the brain. Jon fared poorly at school and despite being in a special needs class, was unable to acquire the expected knowledge. He repeated several school years but by the age of ten, he still had an intellectual age of seven. By thirty he had a job but still lived with his parents. At thirty-one, he was also dependent on written directions to get himself to and from work, a train journey he's made hundreds of times. He's extremely vague when answering questions about his childhood and upbringing, and to help him his parents have compiled photo albums documenting his life and the things he's done, which they go through with him time and time again. Jon really appreciates his albums, but they have a minimal effect on his memory.

Children's long-term memory is particularly interesting but also contradictory. On the one hand, we see that children have a unique learning capacity; they seem to learn new things much more quickly than adults and are able to absorb twenty new words a day already by the age of two. On the other hand, we trust a six-year-old's memories of the last family holiday less than we do her mother's. And how do we reconcile the picture of the learning child with the fact that most of us have no memories at all of our first years of life?

How and why does a child's long-term memory develop? What factors contribute to a better memory, and what factors lead, as in Jon's case, to memory problems that affect both a person's education and life circumstances? Can we, by studying children's memories, learn something about how our sluggish adult learning faculties can somehow be rejuvenated?

CHILDREN'S LONG-TERM MEMORY

Scientific studies confirm this paradoxical aspect of children's memories: children perform at least as well as adults on some

types of memory test, but on others they don't. Take facial recognition, a very simple test of long-term memory. In such a test,
subjects might have to look at twelve portraits, one at a time; a
few minutes later, the photographs are shuffled with twelve new
portraits, upon which the subjects have to look at the set of photographs again and state simply whether they recognize the face.
When three- to five-year-olds do this test, they are able to recognize ninety-eight percent of them, the same hit rate as adults
attain. The conclusion we can draw is that when it comes to simple tests of recognition, children's ability quickly matures to adult
levels.[1]

Most people will know the game *Memory* (or *Concentration*), and
this has also been used to compare the memories of adults and
ten-year-old children. In one study, a pack of twenty cards (ten
pairs of identical images) was spread out face down on a table,
and subjects duly took it in turns to turn over two cards. If the
pictures didn't match, the subjects had to turn the cards back
over and remember the design on the faces in order to try to score
a match on their next turn.

Ten different pictures, associated with twenty different positions, is much more than we are able to retain in working memory
for several minutes. We therefore have to employ the long-term
memory for this task, a task on which ten-year-olds were found to
outperform twenty-year-olds. This result is thus the polar opposite of what we've observed for working memory, where the much
higher capacity is enjoyed by the twenty-year-olds.[2,3]

Eyewitness studies, on the other hand, confirm that children are
not always reliable when it comes to recounting events. The main
problem is that they tend to fill in details from their own imagina-
tions and uncritically insert prompts implied by their interroga-
tors.[4] They also have a lack of insight into their own mnemonic
faculties. In one illustrative case from a study of children's' memory, a five-year-old was given a list of twenty words and asked how
many he thought he'd be able to recall. "All of them," he quickly
replied. After he had duly tried to remember the words, the test
leader pointed out to him that he had only recalled less then half
the list. But he would have another chance with twenty new words.

How many did he think he would be able to recall this time? "All of them," the boy replied again without blinking an eye.

One explanation for these contradictory results is that the long-term memory is not a uniform faculty. The first distinction we must make is between the *encoding* and *retrieval* of memories. Even though both encoding and retrieval are two aspects of what we call "memory," they obey different laws and, as we shall see, involve different parts of the brain. Both encoding and retrieval are affected by a wide range of factors, but not necessarily in the same way. For example, as we will discover in Chapter 8, extreme stress induces better encoding but worse retrieval of long-term memories.

Differences in how well individuals manage to store a memory depend not only on how easy it is to make things "stick" ("sticky memory" versus "Teflon memory") but also on the use of encoding strategies. One of the most critical factors of memory storage is the ability to associate new memories with earlier ones. If we ask someone to look at a number of pictures and ask the person to assess a particular quality of each object, such as whether it can be eaten or worn, his or her memory of the pictures will be much better than if we'd simply asked if there was, say, anything green in them. This phenomenon is referred to as "levels of processing," and it is possibly the outcome of how the analysis of an object's function demands a level of information processing that, in going deeper than simple image recognition, enables associations to be made with previously stored memories.

Children's mnemonic capacity differs according to the type of memory task being performed. But despite the fact that the long-term memory is more like a family of functions and susceptible to a wide range of external and internal factors, there is one area of the brain that is integral to the "stickiness" of long-term memory: the hippocampus.

THE KEY TO THE MEMORY

Scientists first learned of the vital role played by the hippocampus in 1953 following a bilateral hippocampal resection that surgeons carried out at Hartford Hospital in Connecticut in an attempt to cure a particularly severe case of epilepsy. After his operation, the patient, one Henry Molaison (widely known by his initials H. M.), was no longer able to store new memories about his life and was completely unable to recognize the neuropsychologist who would meet him several times a week to test his memory. However, Henry could remember previous life memories and performed perfectly well on certain tests. One such test that the neuropsychologist had Henry do was to trace the contours of a star with a pencil concealed by a screen and only visible to him in a mirror, so that when he pulled the pencil toward him it looked like he was pushing it away, and vice versa. Everyone who performs this test improves with each day of practice. The surprising result of Henry's test was that he also improved just as quickly.

The effects of the operation and the effects that it had on H. M. showed that the encoding of memories is dependent on a small, well-defined brain structure—the hippocampus—but one that is not responsible for the retrieval of old memories or, as Henry's case revealed, for motor learning. From this, we may conclude that there are different types of long-term memory, each related to different parts of the brain (see Fig. 4.1).

The memory function affected by Henry's operation was the encoding of what came to be called *declarative memories*, which are the memories of which we are aware, such as the events we experience or the facts we learn. Some psychologists also divide the declarative memory into *episodic memory*, which encodes the personal experiences, and the *semantic memory*, which encode the facts, as well as the meaning of words and general knowledge that cannot be associated with a specific time and place of learning.

The motor memory, which was not affected by the removal of H. M.'s hippocampus, is a form of unconscious or implicit memory, like the ability to ride a bike or play a musical instrument. Clive, who we met at the start of this chapter, could still play the piano despite his extremely poor declarative memory. The presence of different memory systems in the brain doesn't only

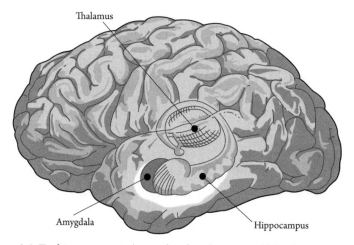

Figure 4.1 The hippocampus is situated within the temporal lobe close to the amygdala, and it plays a critical part in the encoding of long-term memories.

mean that lesions can affect one and leave others intact; it also means that different systems can develop independently during childhood.

Henry Molaison died in 2009 at the age of eighty, after a lifetime of psychological studies and interviews. At one interview toward the end of his life he was asked what he thought when he looked at his reflection in a mirror. He replied, "I'm not a boy."[5]

The maturation principles governing the hippocampus are similar in many respects to those of other parts of the cortex: an early increase in the number of neurons during prenatal growth, a proliferation of synapses and connections after birth, and then a pruning of superfluous branches. This said, compared with the prefrontal cortex, the hippocampus matures relatively early (see Fig. 4.2). The number of synapses reaches a peak at roughly the age of two, and the subsequent pruning is probably completed at around the age of four or five.[6] There is not, however, full scientific consensus here, and some neurologists believe that the hippocampus doesn't reach full maturity until the age of eight. Whichever is the case, it's still earlier than the prefrontal cortex, which continues to thicken up to the age of eleven or twelve, with the pruning effect lasting into the early twenties.

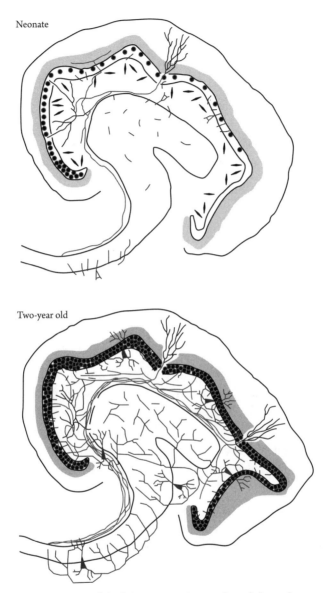

Figure 4.2 The maturity of the hippocampus in a newborn baby and a two-year-old (after Richmond and Nelson, 2007).

The hippocampus differs in one essential respect from most other brain areas: what was once considered a fundamental principal of cerebral development—that no new neurons form after birth—doesn't seem to apply to the hippocampus. More and more data have been produced in recent years showing that new nerve cells form in the hippocampus throughout our lives.*

Cell formation in the hippocampus is more than just an academic curiosity; it's also important for its function. The new neurons link up with the existing ones, creating a matrix that animal studies show affects the long-term memory: the more new cells, the better the encoding into long-term memory. Intensive learning also seems to impact on the survival of these newly formed cells, as has been observed in animals trained to remember a path through a maze. More cells are formed in young individuals than adult ones, and the formation of new hippocampal cells in children and adolescents could be one factor shaping how the "stickiness" trajectory of the long-term memory changes over time.[7]

The child's brain also differs from the adult's at the lowest level, too, in the receptors that receive neurotransmitters and that are active in memory creation. The mechanisms here are complex and take some patience to grasp. Long-term memories are created through the creation or reinforcement of neuronal connections, which are formed when an axon from one neuron extends and opens a synaptic channel of communication with another neuron, but there are a great many preceding neuronal processes. Noted American neurobiologist Eric Kandel, who received the Nobel Prize in Medicine in 2000 for his discoveries of many mnemonic

---

* A confession might be in order here: my account of the hippocampus and the long-term memory is misleadingly simplified. The hippocampus is merely one of several adjacent structures inside the temporal lobe, and it comprises a number of substructures possessing complementary functions. In H. M.'s case, the lesion included not only the hippocampus but also the surrounding structures, which together should more accurately be referred to as the "medial temporal lobe." There is not enough space here to go into detail about the different parts of the medial temporal lobe, and I will continue to use the word *hippocampus* when it would in fact be more correct to write "the hippocampus and adjoining structures of the medial temporal lobe." As regards the formation of new nerve cells in the hippocampus, it is specifically the *gyrus dentatus* where this phenomenon occurs. The maturation rate of the constituent parts of the hippocampus also varies.

mechanisms, observed how primitive memories could be generated by the repeated stimulation of the gigantic nerve cells of a
sea slug.

One of the most important components of memory is the
NMDA receptor, a receptor being a structure on the surface of a
nerve cell that receives signal substances from other nerve cells.
This receptor is made up of a number of proteins, which scientists
have discovered can take different forms, each with its own degree
of effectiveness. In one study on mice, scientists managed to create individuals with more efficient long-term memory encoding
by increasing the amount of one of these proteins (NR2B).[8] An
interesting finding from a developmental perspective is that not
only do the relative amounts of the different proteins change as
we grow up, but this mnemonically beneficial protein is more
prevalent in childhood than it is in adulthood, something that
could be yet another reason why children have a more "sticky"
long-term memory.

Why we don't remember the first years of life remains a mystery.
Sigmund Freud had, as usual, the most fascinating and complex
explanation for our hazy memories of early infancy. According
to Freud, we repress early childhood memories because they are
traumatic and associated with primitive drives; unfortunately,
however, it's a model that has little empirical support. According
to another hypothesis, "infant amnesia" occurs because babies
have no linguistic tags to attach to their memories. Personally,
I've never bought this argument either. My memories of events
and places are very rarely accompanied by verbal descriptions;
images, emotions, and smells require no words, and after all,
mice, apes, and elephants have a fully functional hippocampus
and an ability to create lasting long-term memories despite not
having the gift of speech. Unfortunately, a really good study on
infant pachyderm amnesia is yet to be published.

Another hypothesis that has been forwarded to explain the
lack of early memories is that children don't have a developed
sense of self-identity that enables them to classify memories
later on as being from their own childhood. Again, it's hard to
find any empirical support for this hypothesis. Identity is an

elusive concept and not easy to quantify in experimental studies. However, the link between long-term memory and the experience of a self—a consciousness—is interesting. Perhaps the converse it true: that the long-term memory is essential to the creation of an identity. The diary entries of Clive Wearing, who we met earlier and whose virus infection erased previous memories, believed he had not previously been conscious. How does the gradual development of children's declarative memories shape their identity and consciousness?

For want of other powerful theories of childhood amnesia, we must stick to simple facts about brain development that can explain at least part of the phenomenon. The memory system requires its maturity, just like other parts of the brain. It doesn't seem unreasonable to suppose that the hippocampus should require several years of synaptic growth before it works well enough to create lifelong memories.

So the hippocampus is essential to one specific mnemonic component: the encoding of declarative long-term memories. But in order to create the long-term memories that we use every day it has to integrate with a number of other brain structures. While encoding is initially performed by the hippocampus, it is gradually transferred to parts of the occipital and temporal cortices (see Fig. 2.3 in Chapter 2), and once the memories have been thus transferred, there they remain, even if the hippocampus is damaged—as the case of Henry Molaison, who still remembers his childhood, illustrates. However, if the new memory areas are damaged, as in the case of Clive Wearing and his virus infection, earlier encoded memories are lost as well.

The hippocampus and the temporal cortex have connections with the prefrontal cortex, which plays an important part in the interpretation of sensory impressions and their association with previous knowledge. When we think, reason, and associate around a certain memory, we reinforce that memory: a "levels of processing" effect that greatly aids recall. Memory retrieval also often resembles a problem-solving task: we are given a piece of a puzzle, say a picture of a face, and we search the memory for the context in which we have seen that face (and for a name to go with it, hopefully). Keeping relevant information in the mind during the search process is very much like what we do when performing a working memory task. Moreover, the areas of the prefrontal cortex that are activated when we retain new information in working memory overlap those involved in the retrieval of long-term memories.

Memory tasks that demand no particularly sophisticated form of strategy, such as answering yes or no to the question of whether you recognize a photograph of a face, are just as easy— if not easier—for eight-year-old children to do as they are for adults. However, if the memory task requires some sort of prefrontal activation for handling strategies, reasoning, or holding information in working memory during a long-term memory search, children underperform teenagers and adults. The total mnemonic performance is dependent upon some kind of interaction between an early maturing hippocampus and a later developing prefrontal cortex.

IMPROVING THE LONG-TERM MEMORY

If only a memory were like a photo that we place in a box to be retrieved when needed. Unfortunately, a memory is more like a picture drawn in sand: it's not a particularly accurate representation of the original and is constantly exposed to the erosive wash of time.

The fading of memory over time was studied by German psychologist Hermann Ebbinghaus back in the 1800s. With Teutonic meticulousness and himself as subject, he learned long lists of meaningless letter combinations and tested his memory at varying intervals of time after the initial learning event. Doing this, Ebbinghaus arrived at his now famous forgetting curve, which plots memory loss against time and demonstrates, rather depressingly, that without information review it takes just a few days to forget roughly eighty percent of what we originally learned. However, memories can be refreshed through review. One review not only allows us to remember more of the information

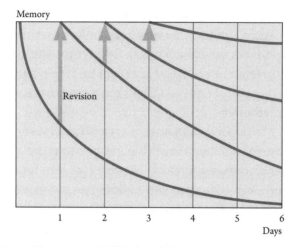

Figure 4.3 An illustration of Ebbinghaus's forgetting curve. Without repetition memory fades quickly. The review of information not only gives better immediate retrieval, it also prevents the information from being forgotten as quickly as it is otherwise would be.

immediately after relearning it but also reduces the steepness of the forgetting curve. A few days after the second learning event we remember roughly forty percent of the information, as opposed to the twenty percent we remember with only the one input phase (Fig. 4.3).

For over a century now, psychologists have been building upon Ebbinghaus's research and have, among other things, worked out the optimal distribution of rehearsal events, developing the "spacing effect" that Ebbinghaus himself had discovered on observing the efficiency gains of spacing out the relearning events over cramming them together tightly.

American psychologist Robert Bjork, UCLA, and others have subsequently shown that the most effective strategy seems to be to gradually spread out periods of rehearsal, so that the first occasion takes place immediately after initial learning with successive relearnings at gradually lengthening intervals.[9] It's likely that the optimal time for rehearsals is when we still remember roughly ninety percent of the input information. It also appears that self-testing is the best way to learn; so if your aim is to memorize a Chinese translation of an English word, it's better to see the

English word and try to remember the Chinese equivalent than it is to passively see the two words presented together.

Piotr Wozniak is a Polish researcher who's made spaced repetition the main principle by which he lives his life. As a student of English and biology, he grew dismayed by how little time there was and how much revision would be needed for him to learn what he wanted to learn. He reasoned that if he distributed his learning more effectively and in accordance with the rules of spacing, he'd be able to achieve his goals much more quickly. The problem, however, was keeping track of what he'd learned and when. So he duly wrote a computer program into which he input the date and content of his study and which would then automatically remind him of when it was time for revision.

The program is now publicly available under the name *SuperMemo* and is sold around the world, mainly as a tool for learning foreign language vocabularies. Piotr himself uses the program to learn not only new words but all kinds of information. He marks the texts or articles he wants to memorize and inputs them in priority order into his software, which then keeps tabs on when it's time for him to refresh his memory. Like Ebbinghaus, Piotr Wozniak uses himself as a subject. So as not to be disturbed by his surroundings when he carries out his lengthy experiments on himself, he carries no mobile phone, answers no e-mails, and can disappear for months to a place where no one can reach him. His lifestyle also includes daily dips in the sea, year round, and never resisting the impulse to sleep.[10]

As interesting a phenomenon as the spacing effect is, the history of its research is a sad example of how poor the communication flow is between psychology, pedagogy, and neuroscience. The advantages of the effect are obvious: by distributing learning events for school or university students, teachers would be able to raise their level of knowledge without extending their time of study. The practical implications of these findings were pointed out by psychologists already in the early 1900s, but despite this their impact on educational theory and practice has been minimal. Indeed, it has even been called one of the twentieth century's most neglected psychological discoveries. With this in mind, one might give up all hope of the possible practical applications of all ongoing research into the psychology of memory.

Nor has the spacing effect benefited from any cross-fertilization between neuroscience and psychology. Kandel's studies on repeated stimulation and long-term memory ignored the spacing effect, and Bjork probably never read a single word on Kandel's sea slugs.

Finding the optimal timetable for the revision of new knowledge is an extremely time-consuming endeavour. One of Bjork's studies from the 1970s included data from 700 people and concluded that a time interval between rehearsals of 1-4-10 is better than 5-5-5. But might 1-2-12 be better? To find out, we'd need another 700 people and two more years of research.

The neurobiology of long-term memory encoding is understood in extreme detail, from the current curves of the NMDA receptors to individual molecular changes in the cellular signal pathways and electron-microscopic images of synapse formation in the hippocampus. Somewhere in all this lurks the explanation for the spacing effect. If neurobiologists took an interest in the spacing effect, they would probably find the principles governing revision effects more quickly and accurately, thus sparing psychologists another century of plying university students with vocabulary lists to learn at different repetition intervals. And then, once these principles have been found, it would be left to the pedagogists to incorporate them into teacher training programs and the school curriculum.

As we have seen, the long-term memory is a family of functions involving different parts of the brain. But the function of the hippocampus is unique. In evolutionary terms, this seahorse-shaped structure is an ancient part of the brain that is set apart not only in the way that it creates new neurons but also in how its early development is particularly sensitive to oxygen deprivation. That was the cause of Jon's problem. When a team of researchers in London led by neuropsychologist Faraneh Vargha-Khadem ran a magnetic resonance scanner over Jon's brain, they found that the lack of oxygen he suffered during birth caused a highly localized contraction of the cortex just around the hippocampus.[11]

The damage wasn't great: only a few square centimeters of his entire cerebral cortex was a few millimeters thinner than normal. But it was enough to profoundly shape Jon's life. Just as his memory problems screen him off from his past, they also seem to render him blind to the future. Visions and plans are things we build and model internally; but memories of actual events and experiences are the stuff of which our future dreams are made. Once when asked what he envisaged his future might be, Jon hesitantly replied: "I have no picture as such."[12]

CHAPTER 5

✧

Mathematics, Memory, and Space

Plato once wrote that mathematics exists in the world of ideas, independent of humankind. The question is how this abstract thing called mathematics is represented in the three-pound grayish-brown clump of cells that fills our skulls. We've seen in Chapter 2 that the brain's maturity can explain improvements in working memory, but how are we to understand the strong links with math? Our knowledge of how the brain represents and processes mathematical concepts comes from analyses of brain activity, studies of children with mathematical difficulties, and case descriptions of exceptionally gifted individuals, like that of Daniel Tammet.

Daniel was born in east London in 1979, the first child of impoverished parents, who would go on to have another eight sons and daughters. Daniel's parents were quick to note that their son was different to their other offspring: he engaged in repetitive behavior, such as banging his head against the wall or spinning a coin for hours on end. He had poor contact with the other children at his nursery and could sit staring at grains of sand while everyone else was running around playing. He was also obsessed with routines and would insist that his parents take him on exactly the same route to his nursery every day. Later, his parents would learn that many of these symptoms were typical of autism, and when he reached adulthood Daniel was diagnosed with Asperger's syndrome. Typical for someone with Asperger's is the display of autistic traits, such as poor social skills and difficulties understanding another person's feelings, and a fixation on monotonous activities, as well as high intellectual faculties.

At the age of four, Daniel began to suffer epileptic fits. In his autobiography, entitled *Born on a Blue Day*, he described the first incident, which was particularly serious and almost fatally deprived him of oxygen, as "an experience unlike any other, as though the room around me was pulling away from me on all sides, and the light inside it leaking out and the flow of time itself coagulated and stretched out into a single lingering moment." At roughly the same age his parents started to notice his fascination with numbers and his exceptional ability to multiply and divide.[1]

Thanks to his good general intellectual and verbal skills, Daniel was able to describe how his feel for numbers was associated with visual images, which gives us unique insight into how an exceptional mathematical genius can take form. He describes himself as having a special visual image or sensation for all numbers up to 10,000. "Five is a clap of thunder or the sound of waves crashing against rocks. Thirty-seven is lumpy like porridge, while 89 reminds me of falling snow." When dividing two numbers, he visualizes spirals, or fractals, spinning downward. This enables him to "see" a division like 13/97 and give the correct answer to a hundred decimal places. When multiplying 53 by 131, the solution (6,943, of course!) appears as a geometric form uniting the two factors.

Daniel was able to use his ability to visualize numbers as an aid for memorizing them more easily, and he beat the European record for recalling the most digits of pi. At his record attempt, which was arranged at a charity event for the National Society for Epilepsy, it took him over five hours to recite the sequence of 22,514 decimals that he'd committed to memory.

Even if people with autism are often drawn to monotonous activities, one can wonder how much fun it was to spend three months memorizing over 20,000 decimals. One of the highlights of Daniel's achievement was reciting the 762nd to the

767th digits, which are 999999. The sequence is called the Feynman point, after the eccentric physicist Richard Feynman, who wanted to learn how to memorize all the digits up to this sequence so that when reciting them aloud he'd be able to end by saying "999999 and so on." "The Feynman point is visually very beautiful to me," wrote Daniel. "I see it as a deep, thick rim of dark blue light."

Daniel also had a special gift for languages, for which he'd use his own vocabulary-learning system. He's said to have learned Icelandic in ten days, and he now masters nine other languages thanks to this same method; he has even invented his own language, which he calls *mänti* after the Finnish word for pine tree. Daniel fared well at school but found it hard to find a job afterward, a fate he shares with many other people with Asperger's. However, owing to his remarkable faculty for languages he can make a living working for an online language school, where he teaches his special system.

Even though Daniel's abilities are unique, his descriptions paint an interesting picture of how numbers are represented visually: in two dimensions along a ruler or in three-dimensional space, which can be a more general cerebral number-manipulation phenomenon. Most children use their fingers when they first learn to count (hence the word *digit*), and in some cultures, counting continues along the arm: the wrist is six, the elbow 7, the shoulder 8, and so on. There are languages in New Guinea that assign the identical word to the body part and the number, so that the word for the left nipple, say, is the same as that for the number 9. This is a practical way of making room for more numbers on the body, but it isn't as good an introduction to the decimal system as the fingers.

Even when a child has left behind the concrete finger-math, he or she still possesses a visual image of numbers. So that now, if you're to solve the sum 11 minus 3, you'll probably still have a vague impression that you're visualizing a kind of number line, or "mental ruler," along which you take three steps back from 11 to give you an answer that you can read off. Psychological studies show that more than being just a side phenomenon, the image of a mental ruler tells us something about how the brain represents numbers with the aid of a visual, spatial image.

In one study, subjects were presented with the numbers 1 to 9 and asked to say if the number they saw was greater or less than 5. If the number was smaller, they had to press a button with one hand; if it was larger, they were to press a button with the other hand. It's a known phenomenon that people react more quickly to images in the left visual field with the left hand, and images in the right visual field with the right hand. This is because impressions from the left visual field are led to the right brain hemisphere and that the same hemisphere also controls the left hand. It turned out that subjects were on average faster with their left hand for the lower numbers and with their right hand for the higher numbers. Despite the fact that our Arabic numerals are abstract symbols and that they were presented to them in the middle of their visual field, the subjects reacted as if the lower numbers were objects that appeared in their left visual field and the higher numbers in the right.[2] The image of a mental ruler is thus not just an association we make as we calculate the solution to a sum; it also seems to be used for the actual calculation, whereby we place numbers along the ruler and then read off the answer.

Furthermore, the time it takes people to ascertain the relative magnitude of two numbers depends on how great the difference between them is. Even though it's obvious that 8 is less than 9, it takes subjects slightly longer to determine this fact than if asked whether 7 is less then 9.[3] A computer would be just as quick at responding in both cases; the human brain, however, seems to take a detour, along which the numbers are converted to positions on a mental ruler, which then has to be inspected, and the closer the numbers are along this visualized line, the longer it takes to discern their relative size. As we shall see later on in this chapter, visualization problems can, in fact, lead to an inability to manipulate numbers. We'll also see how the visualization of objects can form part of a cognitive chain linking working memory and mathematics. But first, let's go back to the beginning and look at how numbers are conceptualized by babies.

COUNTING BABIES

The fact that there's a natural tendency to represent numbers on a mental ruler ought to mean that it's a natural way of teaching numeracy to children. However, this isn't always the case. I'm certainly not alone in having been forced to endure endless hours arranging boxes in order of size and circling sets in a set theory book to develop an "understanding of numbers." Much mathematics teaching has been inspired by the writings of French child psychologist Jean Piaget, and his influence is still felt to this day—even if the teaching of math occasionally involves computers and touch-sensitive screens instead of the flannel board that I was tormented with.

Piaget was originally a biologist, but he soon migrated into the field of psychology. He conducted the bulk of his studies, which often involved a combination of interviews and psychological tests, in the first half of the 1900s, and used his findings to develop theories of the stages of child development. Each phase is characterized by a specific faculty and conception of the outside world, and it is their continual readjustment of this conception through interaction with the world that propels children from stage to stage. Piaget argued that children are unable to understand numbers and their significance until the age of seven, once they have passed through the sensorimotor and preoperational stages, during which they spend years integrating with their surroundings, ideally by comparing blocks, in order to develop an understanding of what a number is and the difference between "two" and "three." We now know that Piaget got it totally wrong.

One of the key experiments that convinced Piaget of the infant's inability to understand numbers concerned something called "number conservation." For this study, the experimenter placed on a table in front of him two equally spaced rows of six glasses and six bottles, and asked his child subjects whether there were more glasses or more bottles, upon which they would usually reply that the amounts were the same. When the spacing was changed so that the row of glasses was longer than the row of bottles and the question was repeated, the children would point to the row of glasses. Not until the age of seven do children generally reply that the rows are still the same, which Piaget took to indicate that it's only then that the human brain has developed an understanding of the concept of number.

However, in 1967, Jacques Mehler and Tom Bever, then of the Massachusetts Institute of Technology, showed that if the bottles and glasses are exchanged for sweets and the children are simply asked to choose which row of sweets they want to eat, they demonstrate a highly advanced understanding of number.[4] If a short row of eight sweets is placed beside a long row of six sweets, even two-year-olds choose the row containing the largest number rather than the longest. It seems that the explanation isn't that reward improves performance. It also seems that Piaget's error has something to do with the artificiality of the situation and the manner in which the questions were asked. Put yourself in a five-year-old's shoes: in front of you are two rows containing an equal number of glasses and bottles. An adult then asks you which row has the most items and then moves some of the glasses and repeats the question. It's obvious to you that the number of glasses and bottles hasn't changed; you've been able to work that out since the age of two. But why is this adult person asking such a silly question? It has to be a trick. Or does this person mean something else by the word "number"? "Best to answer as I'm expected to," the child probably thinks.

In one creative variant of this test carried out by developmental psychologists James McGarrigle and Margaret Donaldson of the University of Edinburgh, the experimenter used a "naughty teddy" glove puppet as an accomplice.[5] The experimenter lined up two rows containing equal numbers of marbles on a table in front of the child. After the experimenter asked the child which row had the most marbles, he would turn away, giving time for the teddy to pop out of its box to rearrange the marbles. The experimenter would then turn back and say to the child something like, "Oh, no, that naughty teddy has messed things up again! Which row has the most marbles now?" In this situation, children were able to differentiate between the number of marbles in a row and its length, while the same children would fail when the experiment was conducted along the lines of Piaget's model.

Later studies have shown that an understanding of number exists already in early infancy. It's not easy to study number sense in neonates as they can neither answer questions nor point. However, some rather elegant studies have successfully used subtle behaviors, such as gaze direction and dummy-sucking intensity, to unravel what's going on in the baby's brain.

When babies are shown the same picture a repeated number of times, they look at it for ever shorter lengths of time. If the picture is replaced by a different one, they will demonstrate revived interest by spending more time looking at the picture and sucking more intensively on their dummies. By measuring dummy sucking and eye movements, researchers are able to determine what a baby perceives as a new object. With the application of this method, it's possible to show that babies can already perceive whether a picture contains one, two, or three objects just a few days after birth.[6] If babies are shown repeated pictures of the same number of objects, say three cars, three balls, or three bottles, they eventually lose interest. However, if the pictures are exchanged for ones depicting two objects, children become surprised and look at them for longer. Control experiments also demonstrated that this had nothing to do with the appearance of the pictures, only the number of objects. So as early as just a few days after birth, children have a conception of number—at least up to three.

How early does the ability to add appear? In one study of five-month-old babies, researchers used a puppet theatre with a screen in the middle of the stage.[7] A hand holding a puppet would enter stage left and hide it behind the screen. The hand would then enter a second time with a new puppet, which would also be placed behind the screen. The screen would then be lowered to reveal the two previously hidden puppets. The procedure would then be repeated but this time with the addition of a trapdoor, through which a puppet could be removed or added; so that when lowered, the screen would reveal not two puppets, as the audience would have been expecting, but either one or three. When

1 + 1 thus equaled 1 or 3, the children looked for much longer than when 1 + 1 equaled 2. This shows that even five-month-old babies not only have a working memory that enables them to remember what's behind the screen; they also have the ability to use this faculty to add up.

RETAINING NUMBERS IN WORKING MEMORY

Pooh was sitting in his house one day, counting his pots of honey, when there came a knock on the door. "Fourteen," said Pooh. "Come in. Fourteen. Or was it fifteen? Bother. That's muddled me."

—From *The House at Pooh Corner*, Chapter 3

In some instances, the relationship between counting and memory is obvious. In our study of children in Nynäshamn, we found that working memory capacity correlates highly with performance in a test of mathematics (see Chapter 1). Almost half of the difference between individuals was attributable to differences in working memory. Visuospatial working memory also determined how the children's mathematical performance changed over time, and those children with better working memories made greater progress in math from one test session to the next two years later; no such correlation was found, however, between long-term memory or reading and mathematical skills.[7a]

The relationship that exists between normal variations in working memory and math also applies to individuals with pronounced difficulties in the subject. In one study, Susan Gathercole at York University identified children who performed more than two standard deviations below the mean on mathematical tests, placing them among the lowest performing two percent.[8] The children carried out a number of working memory tests and their results were compared with children without difficulties. What Gathercole found was a distinct working memory impairment in children with poor mathematical skills. That their difficulties were pronounced for both visuospatial and verbal working memory but not for verbal short-term memory (which is the ability to retain information through silent repetition, like when we run a door code or a telephone number around in our minds until we've punched in the right sequence) ought to indicate some aberration either in the parietal or frontal areas that are activated by working memory tasks but that are not involved in verbal short-term memory.

The visuospatial working memory is closely related to reasoning and fluid intelligence, which is the ability to find connections and draw conclusions independent of previous knowledge. An alternative explanation for the ties between working memory and math would be that intelligence affects both faculties. If this was so, one might expect to observe a statistical relationship between working memory and math that obeys no direct causality. To be sure, it is true that fluid intelligence has an influence on mathematical skills, but we, like other researchers, have shown that working memory still has a significant part to play even when the intelligence effect is statistically controlled for.[9] In our study, working memory was also a stronger predictor of mathematical development than fluid intelligence.

But how can we explain the strong relationship between math and working memory? Perhaps working memory is needed to remember all the intervening stages of a calculation that requires a sequence of operations. For example, the easiest way of multiplying 6 by 13 is to multiply 6 by 10, which gives 60, multiplying 6 by 3, which gives 18, and then adding the two sums together to get 78. The question "6 x 13" and the results of the intervening operations ("60" and "18") must be retained in working memory if we're to arrive at the correct solution; which is one explanation for why working memory is needed for solving mathematical problems.

Research on the mental ruler provides another, perhaps even more important, explanation. Retaining an inner, visual and spatial representation of something is exactly what the visuospatial working memory is there for. It's likely that the same system that keeps information on different positions in working memory also retains the image of the mental ruler. To find out whether this is the case, we need to look a little more closely at which areas of the brain are actually activated when solving a mathematical problem.

THE MNEMONIC MAP

In *The Number Sense*, Stanislas Dehaene describes a patient, referred to as M, who was afflicted by an inability to add and subtract.[10] M had suffered a stroke that initially affected both his speech and movements, but eventually his motor problems receded, and in conversation with Stanislas he appeared completely normal. M could also read words and numbers, but when he was tested on a battery of mathematical tasks, his problems grew more manifest. Asked which number lies between 3 and 5, he'd first reply 3, then 2; asked what lies between 10 and 20, he'd reply 30. M was fluent in his recital of the times tables ("nine times three is twenty-seven" etc.) but that seemed to be knowledge stored in his long-term memory more than the result of repeated addition. He could perform some additions with units for which the sum was less than 10, but this was also conceivably due to long-term memory recall. When the sum was higher than 10, he'd run into severe difficulties; while subtraction was even harder. When asked, "What's 9 minus 8?" he'd answer "7" and would insist that 3 minus 1 was 4.

When M's brain was examined with a magnetic resonance (MR) scanner, it was found that his stroke had caused a major lesion in his parietal lobe. So it's around here that we should be looking for his inability to compare numbers and subtract. But the parietal lobe is a large area, and it's only recently that scientists have been able to study brain activity to localize with any precision the areas responsible for number sense.

Oliver Simon and Stanislas Dehaene at Inserm in Orsay, France, studied the brain activity of subjects as they viewed numbers from 2 to 9, subtracted the number they saw from 11, and said the answer quietly to themselves.[11] The control task involved similar silent self-repetition but with letters. The calculation task activated a well-defined area of the cortex lying in one of the largest furrows in the parietal lobe called the intraparietal sulcus. These results substantiated a number of previous studies showing how injuries around the parietal lobe create problems in number sense. The authors of the study also linked back to studies of monkeys in which scientists had found that the parietal lobe contains neurons that code for specific numbers, so that one neuron would fire if the monkey was shown one object but not two, another if the monkey was shown two objects but not one or three.[12] Several scholars, including Stanislas Dehaene, therefore contend that there is a small area of the intraparietal cortex that only represents number, regardless of whether the number relates to viewed objects or read numerals.

The area of the intraparietal cortex is interesting because it's the very place that several studies have shown is activated when someone retains visuospatial information in working memory. In the Nynäshamn study, we also analyzed what kind of brain activity was associated with a better visuospatial working memory. The psychological tests included measures of the quantity of information each child was able to keep in his or her working memory—that is, how many items each child was able to remember before error started to creep in. The brain activity of over eighty children was then measured while they carried out a visuospatial working memory task in the MR scanner. We found the strongest relationship, not surprisingly, in the intraparietal cortex, in the very same area that was activated when people carried out subtraction tasks in Simon and Dehaene's study: children with higher activity in this area displayed a more effective visuospatial working memory. Moreover, the activity in this region could also predict how much the children would improve in math over the coming two years.[13]

Let's now take a look at the mechanisms responsible for working memory to help us understand how these results fit together. If I ask you to remember exactly where you've seen an object, the constant activity of the nerve cells that code for this particular position will keep the information in working memory. If the activity is interrupted, the memory vanishes. Different nerve cells code for different positions, so that one cell is active if you've seen something diagonally to your upper right, while another would have been active if you'd seen it to your left. The neurons of the intraparietal cortex thus create a two-dimensional mnemonic map. A similar such map exists in the frontal lobe near the area that controls eye movement. The map is not an exact representation of what you've seen but part of the brain system that keeps tabs on *where* you've seen something. Other parts analyze *what* you've seen, like colors and movements.

Numbers are obviously rendered in the brain in analog form, with low numbers to the left and high ones to the right, as though we had a mental ruler on which a number is represented as a point or position. In cultures reading from the right to the left, the number line tends to go in the other direction, but it is still a spatial representation, and that is the point. If we accept that the brain is equipped with the ability to create a mnemonic map, an ability that's probably so ancient that it's even found in primates, it's logical to assume that the same mechanisms are also used to represent positions along a mental ruler. The mnemonic map and the mental ruler would thus reside in the same brain area. A mnemonic map in the parietal cortex would at least explain one of the direct associations between working memory and mathematics.

There are other interesting links between number sense and working memory. The number four seems to be a critical capacity limit that recurs in both areas. Even in infancy we have an ability to retain three to four objects in working memory, which lends credence to the notion of some innate capacity limit in the parietal mnemonic map. As adults we can use the prefrontal cortex to stretch this capacity to around seven units, but in working memory tasks in which the repetition of information is prevented, the capacity limit for the parietal cortex is still four units. It also turns out that four is also the limit to our ability to immediately perceive number. If you see a flock of birds take to the air from a bush, you'd be roughly just as quick at ascertaining their number if there were one, two, three, or four birds. Computerized tests reveal that when the number exceeds four, reaction times increase by about 250 milliseconds per object. This is a well-documented phenomenon that suggests that the brain can immediately recognize up to four objects; any more, and we have to start counting them one by one, our reaction time rising linearly with number. It might be just coincidence, but this could have something to do with an in-built capacity limit in the parietal mnemonic map that affects both working memory and number sense.

In *Rain Man*, Dustin Hoffman portrays a person with autistic traits but also a unique faculty for memory and for mental arithmetic—in other words, a *savant* not unlike Daniel Tammet. In one scene, a waitress drops a box of toothpicks on the floor. Hoffman's character (Raymond) mumbles "82, 82, 82 ... 246." The waitress reads from the box that it contains 250 toothpicks, but just as Raymond and his brother are leaving the diner, she turns and says: "There's four left in the box."

This episode was probably borrowed from a case study written about by neurologist Oliver Sacks. In his best-selling book *The Man Who Mistook His Wife for a Hat*, he gives an account of a meeting with a pair of twins who are both savants.[14] They have an IQ of 60, which corresponds to serious retardation, but also a particular gift for figures. When Sacks empties a box of matches onto the table, they both immediately exclaim: "111" and then "37, 37, 37." "How did you work that out?" asks Sacks. They didn't work it out, they said, they "saw" it. When he counts the matches, he finds that, sure enough, there are exactly 111 of them.

Oliver Sacks also describes how the twins' favorite hobby was to exchange six-digit prime numbers which they had not memorized but somehow apparently calculated, or rather "saw" as a mental image. While no studies have been made of their brains, it's still exciting to speculate what might lie behind the twins' remarkable abilities. Might it be some aberration of brain development that has happened to give their parietal mnemonic maps an abnormal capacity? This would enable them to sense 37 immediately, the normal capacity being 4. This abnormal mnemonic map could also be the reason for their unique mental arithmetic skills.

MATHEMATICAL AREAS

The intraparietal cortex and its mnemonic map is a link between the visuospatial working memory and number sense, as well as the ability to compare, add, and subtract numbers. But there's much more to mathematics than this, and it's not just the intraparietal cortex that is necessary for solving mathematical problems. The faculty of numeral reading requires the same sort of visual decoding as letter reading, although it resides in other areas of the occipital lobe. Mathematical knowledge stored in the long-term memory, such as the times tables, is more language-related and associated with the lower part of the parietal cortex and frontal lobe. M had problems with subtraction and saying which numbers lie between 10 and 20, but he could recall his times tables, suggesting that these abilities are dependent on different parts of the brain. Interestingly, there are studies of brain lesions that lead to exactly the opposite phenomenon: a loss of times table recall but an unimpaired ability to subtract.[15] With reservations that this is an incomplete map, Figure 5.1 gives an overview of the some of the most critical areas used in mathematical reasoning.

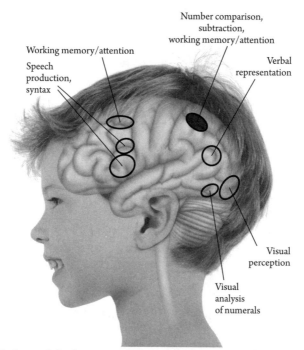

Figure 5.1 Areas of the brain activated on the solving of mathematical problems. The blackened area is the intraparietal cortex, the area associated with dyscalculia (adapted from Dehaene et al., 2004).[16]

The model gives clear predictions of the effects we would expect to see on damage to different parts of the brain: damage to the visual areas of the occipital lobe would lead to an inability to read numerals but leave unaffected calculations of numbers heard instead of seen. Damage to the pathways between the occipital area and the prefrontal cortex would create problems articulating numbers as well as reading difficulties, but it would not affect the ability to multiply or subtract. Damage to the inferior parietal cortex would create problems remembering the times tables but not subtracting. Damage to the intraparietal cortex would create problems representing and comparing numbers and subtracting and adding, but it would not affect information stored in the long-term memory, such as the times tables or sums under 10, which have often been learned by heart.

By "damage" we mean the obliteration of a brain structure by whatever means, such as a stroke as in the case of M. But the link between brain area and function also applies to normal variation. We know very little about how genes shape brain development, but studies of identical twins show that the size of many brain areas is hereditary. If someone happens to have inherited genes that give an above-average number of connections or neurons in the parietal cortex, we would expect it to affect the person's number sense and working memory but not his or her ability to read numerals or learn his or her times tables. So the map of brain functions thus explains the links between individual variations in different abilities. If we return for a moment to the question of what significance cognitive neuroscience has to educational theory and practice, maps like that in Figure 5.1 provide one answer.

Of course, the map cannot be applied to mathematical teaching just like that, but it does illustrate the components of mathematical understanding and explain individual differences in mathematical skills.

MATHEMATICS AND GENDER

In the early 1990s, toy company Mattel launched their Teen Talk Barbie, which would rattle off a selection of phrases at the push of a button: "Do you have a crush on anyone?" was one, "I love shopping!" another. But then there was "Math class is tough." A more blatant example of stereotyped gender roles is hard to find. So what's the real story behind gender differences in math: do they exist?

The gender difference has been documented by several major studies. In 1980, Camilla Persson Benbow and Julian Stanley at Johns Hopkins University published a paper in *Science* with data from almost 10,000 individuals showing that boys of the age of around thirteen or fourteen performed roughly half a standard deviation—which is to say around eight percent—better than girls of the same age.[17] The study was well controlled and the researchers were able to eliminate the possible effect of teaching approaches on performance and other potential influences. Half a standard deviation is also quite a big difference, and it means that only one in three girls performed better than the mean performance of the boys.

However, later studies have shown that the relationships are more complex than this. A paper from 2008 collated the results from a study testing the reading and mathematical literacy of over 250,000 children from around the world (the Program for International Student Assessment, or PISA).[18] The math part of the test included four different disciplines: geometry, algebra, arithmetic, and probability, and the children's scores were aggregated into a "combined mathematics literacy score" for each individual. The results lend some support to the previous American observation, namely that the boys were better than the girls. But the difference was not as great as it was twenty years earlier, and the means were now only a tenth of a standard deviation (roughly 1.5 percent) apart. There was also considerable international variation: in Turkey, the difference was double that of the United States, in Sweden and Norway there was no statistical difference at all, while in Iceland, the girls actually outperformed the boys.

To test the hypothesis that cultural differences could explain these variations, the researchers used the *Gender Gap Index*, an accepted measure of gender differences in society compiled by the autonomous World Economic Forum. The index is based on a range of factors, such as how well women are represented in business, politics, and education, which are pooled to give a total index score that approaches 1 the more equal representation the society has.

What they found was that the *Gender Gap Index* correlated very highly with the gender differences observed in mathematical skills: countries such as Turkey, Korea, and Italy, where the gender gap is the widest, also showed the greatest difference in test achievement. The Nordic countries (Sweden, Norway, and Iceland) had the most widespread equality and the closest performances between the sexes. The researchers also worked out that if all countries were as egalitarian as the Nordics, there would be no differences in mathematical literacy (with the exception of a slight one in geometry), while the gender gap in reading literacy would remain.

However, the study was unable to explain the causality. Why should the number of women in parliament influence a fifteen-year-old girl's mathematical abilities? In Chapter 8 we'll see how this could have something to do with how the brain is affected by stress. Incidentally, Mattel has now updated Barbie's vocabulary.

DYSCALCULIA—DOES IT EXIST?

When the restaurant bill comes and everyone has to chip in, a certain paralysis often descends on the company. The eyes viewing the various sum totals glaze over, not just because of the number of decimal places or the awkwardness of discussing, but because the adding up is just so laborious. Many people hate having to do sums in their head.

Our aptitude for handling numbers follows a normal variation pattern, but for those at the tail end of the curve a diagnosis has been reserved: dyscalculia. The term *dyscalculia* (or developmental dyscalculia) is defined as "a specific learning disability affecting the normal acquisition of arithmetic skills in spite of normal intelligence, emotional stability, scholastic opportunity, and motivation."[19] Pinning down the notion of "disability" can itself be tricky, and scholars have posited a wide range of definitions, from the individual's capacity to be taught to the relativity of mathematical literacy to other cognitive abilities.[20] However, one criterion that's often applied is that the individual in question must perform at least 1.5 standard deviations below the mean while displaying an otherwise normal IQ. With this definition, between three and six percent of all school children qualify for the diagnosis and it's just as common among girls as it is boys.

Even before the term had come into more widespread general use, it was causing conflict. Many people are sceptical about the use of all types of quasi-medical category, be it dyslexia, attention-deficit/hyperactivity disorder (ADHD), or dyscalculia. Others maintain that children who have trouble with math have nothing more complex than general intellectual difficulties and that introducing a separate diagnostic term is irrelevant. Scholars who have long upheld the diagnosis of dyslexia argue that dyscalculia must be seen as a subcategory of dyslexia and that the problem is a fundamentally linguistic one.

It's also true that many of those who'd be diagnosed with dyscalculia would also qualify for the diagnosis of dyslexia and ADHD. However, there are also studies showing that dyslexia and dyscalculia can be disengaged from each other: children with dyscalculia have greater numerical difficulties; children with dyslexia have greater phonological difficulties. In one study, children with either diagnosis were given a battery of working memory tests to perform. It was found that children with dyscalculia had most trouble with their visuospatial working memory, but not with their phonological short-term memory.[21] So visuospatial working memory and math are associated regardless of whether children have been diagnosed with dyscalculia.

Notwithstanding the theoretical and political disagreements about dyscalculia, the term is used in academia and generates knowledge of the relationship between mathematical skills and the brain. One study looked at the brain activity of children with and without dyscalculia as they performed a visuospatial working memory task, and it found that those with dyscalculia showed lower brain activity in the right intraparietal cortex and two regions of the frontal lobes.[22] They also had a lower volume of white matter. Moreover, the activity in the right parietal lobe correlated with how well they performed on two different working memory tests outside the MR scanner.

Another study of children with dyscalculia employed a task that demanded no calculations or numerals, just the appreciation of number.[23] The subjects were shown two sets of squares on a screen and asked to decide which set contained the most: if there were seven squares to the left of the screen and five to the right, they were to press the left button. Children with dyscalculia had trouble with this task, especially when the difference between the two sets was small. When the brain activity of a group with dyscalculia was compared with that of a control group, the researchers observed once again that the dyscalculia group displayed a lower degree of activity in the right intraparietal cortex as well as in two areas of the frontal lobe and occipital lobe.

One area that emerges again and again in studies of dyscalculia is precisely the intraparietal cortex. To specifically ascertain the significance of this region, researchers have also tried to disable the function of the parietal cortex in an attempt to artificially produce symptoms similar to those of dyscalculia. To "disable" a brain area might sound dramatic, but there's no surgery involved. The method used is called transcranial magnetic stimulation and involves placing a 15 cm insulated cable, shaped like a figure eight, around the head. When a current passes through the cable, a magnetic field is produced that disrupts neuronal signaling in an area of the cortex a few square centimeters in dimension. The function of this area is thus disabled for a few seconds (or minutes) while the subject is tested, giving scientists the opportunity to ascertain whether this area is associated with a certain function. When Roi Cohen-Kadosh and colleagues at University College in London disrupted the function of the parietal cortex in this manner, they found that their subjects had difficulty with simple mathematical tasks, such as determining which of two numbers was the higher.[24] In effect, they had created a virtual dyscalculia.

The results obtained by different studies of dyscalculia are remarkably consistent in pinpointing the intraparietal cortex as the critical region. In a review article on dyscalculia from 2009, the authors condense the current scientific situation into one sentence: "Research indicates that developmental dyscalculia involves a single brain area abnormality—in the intraparietal sulcus."[25]

Dyscalculia is largely hereditary.[26,27] One twin study shows that as many as between sixty and seventy percent of mathematical difficulties among seven- to nine-year-olds is genetically conditioned and only ten percent attributable to their environment.[28] The genetic effect exists both for normal variation in mathematical ability and for the risk of dyscalculia. In that the same genetic pattern is observed in the population at large and in those who have specific problems, dyscalculia is interpreted not as a specific disorder but as a term to describe the individuals who happen to have most trouble with math. Roughly half of the individuals with dyscalculia also have reading and writing difficulties. It has been suggested that a more general impairment of the left parietal lobe explains both kinds of difficulty—that is, math and reading—while a more specific impairment of the intraparietal cortex, or only the right parietal lobe, produces dyscalculia without reading problems. But this is still mere conjecture.

PREMATURE BIRTH AND DYSCALCULIA

Besides the normal, inherent variation in mathematical skills, there are several conditions that are associated with a higher risk of dyscalculia, such as epilepsy, Turner's syndrome, the fragile X syndrome, and extremely premature birth. The largest group comprises children who were born extremely prematurely with a low birth weight, a phenomenon that has, moreover, become all the more common as the growing popularity of in vitro fertilization and artificial insemination has increased the number of twin and triplet pregnancies, and improved maternity care has upped the survival rate of extremely premature babies.

In one Australian study, researchers examined a combined group of children who either had a birth weight of less than 1 kg (approximately 2.2 pounds) or who were born before the 28th week.[29] The control group consisted of children born with a normal birth weight and in the normal week of pregnancy. The children were tested at the age of eleven. What they found was that the study group underperformed the controls on a number of functional tests, including tests of language, long-term memory, reaction time, and working memory. However, the most pronounced problems they had were in tests of mathematical ability. Seven percent of the extremely premature children had serious trouble with math, as opposed to only one percent in the control group. Moderate impairment was observed in twenty-six percent of the extremely premature group, compared with eleven percent in the control group. These cognitive difficulties meant that the children born extremely prematurely had to retake a class twice as often as other children, and were twice as often in need of special teaching.

The brains of extremely premature babies have a number of developmental aberrations that might explain their problems. Individual variation is large and the area of the brain affected determines the problems they have. One study looked at a group of teenagers, all of whom had been born extremely prematurely and subsequently diagnosed with dyscalculia.[30] The team analyzed the thickness of their gray matter with an MR scanner and compared it with a control group. It turned out that the study group had thinner layers of gray matter in one particular area: the intraparietal cortex. Many of the children probably had more widespread aberrations in other regions of the brain, but that of the intraparietal cortex was the lowest common denominator in precisely this group, which had been selected for their dyscalculia. The link between the intraparietal cortex and number sense thus applies not only to the normal variation in mathematical ability and children with a congenital risk of dyscalculia but also to mathematical problems related to extremely premature birth.

Most changes in the brain are small and can only be detected by comparing an entire group of children displaying similar problems with another group of problem-free children. Many scientists hope that in the future we'll be able to improve our analytical methods so that small deviations can be discovered even when studying individuals. This would enable the early identification of children at risk of developing cognitive problems long before they emerge in the classroom, so that they can be given the extra support and training they need. Individuals would then be characterized on the basis not of current diagnoses, such as ADHD or dyslexia, but of the region of the brain where some abnormality has been observed. Teachers would then be faced with the question of how best to help a child with "reduced cortical thickness in the right intra and inferior parietal cortex." I daresay that an upgrade of the neuroscientific component of teacher training courses will be necessary.

TRAINING PROGRAMS

Hopefully, this new knowledge about number sense and dyscalculia will feed into new teaching methods. Drs. Anna Wilson and Stanislas Dehaene at Inserm in Orsay, France, the same experimental psychologists that led many of the studies on number sense and the intraparietal cortex, have built a computerized training program based on research into dyscalculia. The program is called *The Number Race* and can be downloaded for free from the Web site of the organization Unicog.[31] The game was also written using open code so that it can be modified and developed. There are versions in Dutch, English, German, Spanish, French, Greek, Finnish, and Swedish. The core of the program is the training of numerical comparison, a task that activates the intraparietal cortex and that people with dyscalculia have major difficulties performing. The tasks are made harder by decreasing the discrepancy between the numbers to be compared. Another central principle of the program is to stimulate the association between number and spatial representation—or the use, in other words, of the intraparietal mental ruler.

In a pilot study, Wilson and her colleagues studied nine children with dyscalculia who, over a period of four to five weeks, spent half an hour a day, four days a week, learning with the program.[32] When the training period was over, the children were found to be quicker at immediate number recognition and at comparing numbers, and better at subtraction. In a later study they used a shorter training period and evaluated the effect on a group of preschool children from socially deprived backgrounds and a control group who'd been given reading skills training. What they discovered was that the children who had used *The Number Race* were better at number comparison when the numbers were presented as numerals or words, but not when presented as items to count. It is possible that the training period was too brief (there were only six sessions) and more studies are needed.

Other researchers have latched on to the principle of the mental ruler. Psychologist Sharon Griffin has devised a pedagogical method called *Number World* to teach mathematics to preschoolers.[33] The point here is to use visual cues that match the spatial representation of numbers, but instead of blocks there are number lines, thermometers, and board games. The method has been evaluated several times with good results. One study showed, for instance, that around fifty percent more children succeeded on a battery of tests, including numerical comparison, after having been taught using *Number World*. A compilation of scientifically supported pedagogical methods for dyscalculia can be found in Brian Butterworth and Dorian Yeo's book *Dyscalculia Guidance: Helping Pupils with Specific Learning Difficulties in Maths.*[34]

Daniel Temmet excels in the very type of mathematical skill that we have seen is dependent on the intraparietal cortex. He also has a unique ability to visualize numbers. What's interesting about his mathematical gift is that it applies specifically to arithmetic, or numerical calculation. Algebra, which involves solving problems that contain letter symbols, such as the equation $9 = 2x + 3$, has always been difficult for him, and he never received top grades in math at school. We can understand why this was the case by returning to the map showing how different mathematical skills are located in different parts of the brain (Fig. 5.1).

Even though Daniel's description can provide some insight into what the mental universe of a savant looks like, we know very little about what it is in his brain that creates these abilities. It's thought that synesthesia, which leads him to associate numbers with images and sounds, is caused by an abnormally strong connection between different parts of the brain that code for the different sensory modalities. In Daniel's case, scholars have speculated that it could have been his epileptic fits that created these abnormal connections, although the reverse causality is also possible: that it was an innate connection pattern that caused the attacks.

Daniel once took part in a brain mapping study that recorded his brain activity while he memorized regular and irregular sequences of numbers.[35] His readings were then compared with those of a control group that had been asked to perform the same tasks. Given how Daniel describes his number-associated images, the researchers expected to see more activity in different parts of the visual cortex. But this is not what they found. Instead, it was Daniel's frontal lobes, both left and right, that were more active. And while distinct differences were found in the control group between regular sequences (2, 4, 6, 8...) and irregular sequences (7, 2, 5, 9, 8...), they were not in Daniel. To him, it seems as if every number is a unique entity, and all sequences equally special. Clearly, this uniqueness also applies to his brain.*

---

* We will be returning to Daniel Tammet and Joshua Foer's comments on his case in Chapter 9.

CHAPTER 6

❧

Reading, Dyslexia, and Problematic Relationships

Pablo Picasso's dyslexia is commonly cited as a reassuring example of how a dysfunction in one area doesn't preclude excellence in another. Unfortunately, the converse is usually the case: problems in one area are very often related to problems in another, a phenomenon sometimes referred to as the Matthew effect: "To all those who have, more will be given."

In Chapter 5, we noted that there was a connection between dyslexia and dyscalculia. Studies differ in their estimates, but between one-third and two-thirds of all children with dyscalculia also have dyslexia.[1,2] There is a similarly strong correlation between attention-deficit/hyperactivity disorder (ADHD) and an increased risk of both dyslexia and dyscalculia, whereby between twenty and forty percent of those who have the one diagnosis also have the other.[3,4] Just how these relationships arise remains something of a mystery, but we can find one clue to the puzzle by looking at how the brain organizes reading and writing. So let us now turn to reading acquisition and the brain areas involved so that we can come a little closer to the crux of dyslexia and to its possible causes.

In the 1980s, neuropsychologist Uta Frith of University College, London, formulated a theory of reading development based on three strategies: (1) logographic; (2) alphabetic; and (3) orthographic.[5] The first stage of reading development is the instant recognition of familiar words that allows a three-year-old to recognize her name above her coat peg at nursery and other important words. But despite Linnea's ability to recognize her own name, spelled out in letters, she has no idea how to pronounce a syllabic fragment of that word, such as "lin." In terms of development, the logographic strategy is a dead end.

The second stage of reading acquisition is when the child has learned the principles of the reading code: characters, either individually or in clusters, represent sounds that can be joined together to form words. Once the child has cracked this code, she's on the right track. Making the link between phonemes (sound units) and the graphemes (letter units) requires the ability not only to identify and differentiate between letters but also to analyze how a series of phonemes form a word. Teaching a child to play with the phonemes of words therefore gives good preparation for future reading skills. Children who are better able to analyze the phonemes of words also learn to read more quickly.

The third strategy identified by Frith is the orthographic. After hundreds of hours of practice, children no longer need to read the phonemes out loud to decode words but can do so at a glance. Reading is automatic and fluent, and children can read short words as quickly as long ones, at least those up to eight letters long.

LEARNING TO READ

Learning to read places many advanced demands on the brain. First of all, we have to develop the ability to immediately recognize small, almost identical abstract symbols comprising a few curved or straight lines. It appears that the brain has cordoned off a special cortical zone for this very purpose, a postage stamp-sized area of the left temporal lobe, squeezed between one specializing in face recognition and another that analyzes object shape, which has come to be called the "letterbox" area. The letterbox area is located in the same place in almost all individuals and is activated whether it's Italian, English, or Chinese that we're reading.

The fact that the brain has a letterbox area that's universally located in the same place is remarkable; it's as if we're born with an inherent capacity for reading. Given that reading is such a distinct cultural phenomenon and that individuals around the world are put through a wide range of learning methodologies, we would expect the brain areas engaged to vary from culture to culture and person to person. French neuroscientist Stanislas Dehaene has proffered the explanation that we are born with a conglomeration of neurons that, by virtue of their connection matrix, are particularly well disposed for analyzing how linear contours, such as Y, T, and L shapes, create images of objects.[8] Without reading acquisition, we would have used this area to analyze outlines, which means that writing has been adapted to suit the brain's built-in faculties. Theoretically this is interesting, since it contradicts the notion of the brain as a tabla rasa that is written upon through interaction with our environment and our culture during childhood. So culture, implies Dehaene, is also formed in accordance with preexisting cerebral conditions.

The letterbox area was originally a contour-recognition area. The difference between object contours and letters is that the identification of the former is not dependent on their orientation. There is a natural classification of contours and objects that takes no account of reflection, so at first it's natural for children to write an E backward and confuse b and d. The equating of reflected objects is a habit that the brain must gradually wean itself off, while the letterbox area is trained to become ever more efficient at identifying letters and combinations of letters.

Brain maps taken of children of different ages and reading abilities show that the activity of the letterbox area is directly associated with reading ability rather than age.[9] Once the letters have been identified, the next step is to link the letterbox area with those that analyze phonemes. Again, it seems that there is a specific part of the temporal lobe, just above the letterbox area, that governs this very task.

The neurological core of reading acquisition is thus a small network consisting of a letterbox area and a phonological area in mutual communication. However, reading a text involves a great

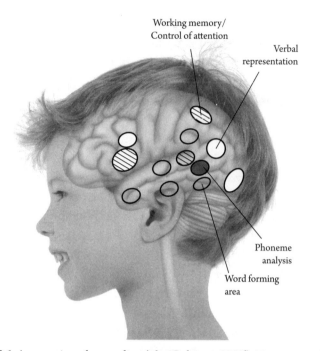

Working memory/
Control of attention

Verbal
representation

Phoneme
analysis

Word forming
area

Figure 6.1 Areas activated on reading (after Dehaene, 2009[8]). The areas marked in white are also activated during mathematical reasoning. The hashed areas are activated during both reading and working memory tasks. The area marked in black is used in the analysis of phonemes. It's a dysfunction of this area that has the strongest association with dyslexia.

many other linguistic functions to keep the reader concentrated on the words and their meaning, enable the reader to remember the beginning of a sentence until he or she has reached the end, associate meanings and connotations to the long-term memory, and link the printed letters to brain areas that deal with their phonic representation and the spoken language. Figure 6.1 shows some of the areas activated in reading. Lack of space prevents me from describing all their respective functions, but some have already been mentioned and it might be worth exploring these connections a little more deeply.

READING AREAS OF THE BRAIN AND DYSLEXIA

If we superimpose the map of reading areas onto that of mathematical areas (see Fig. 5.1 in Chapter 5), we find four structural overlaps. The areas at the back of the occipital lobe and the areas toward the front of the brain are related, respectively, to visual perception and speech production and syntax. Maybe it's not so strange that both the input and output of information is shared by different functions. Another two overlap zones are in the parietal lobe. One is in the lower part and deals with verbal representation and verbal memory, both of which are important for mathematics and reading. Learning the times tables, for example, is verbally based and activates the same parietal areas as reading.

The last overlap zone is in the intraparietal cortex. To complicate the puzzle further, if we superimpose this map with the map of brain areas involved in working memory (see Fig. 2.3 in Chapter 2), we find that the area of the intraparietal cortex isn't only important to reading and math, it's also one of the common working memory areas activated during both verbal and visuo-spatial memory tasks. It is this area that we described in Chapter 5 as the mnemonic map: a blackboard that can be used to keep spatial information in working memory and to remember where in space we have to direct our attention. It's this attention control that is important for reading.

This triple overlap between reading, math, and working memory can be one reason why children with low working memories, such as Nathan in Chapter 1 and Laura in Chapter 2, often have problems with these very skills as well as their ability to concentrate. In our Nynäshamn study, we found that both the verbal and visuospatial working memories of the participants were closely linked to reading comprehension; moreover, British psychologist Susan Gathercole has shown that children with special needs in math and children with the poorest reading comprehension also have greatly impaired working memories,[10] and that if we identify children with reading difficulties but not necessarily dyslexia, we find that working memory is one of the most poorly developed of their cognitive functions.

This commonality of brain area is a possible reason why poor mathematical skills are associated with difficulties in reading and writing. The question is whether it is these very overlapping areas that are the crux of dyslexia. Given the large network of areas needed for reading, it's not surprising that the system can malfunction. Even if we just focus on the core of reading acquisition—the translation from phoneme to grapheme—we would expect to find at least three prime suspects for reading acquisition difficulties in children: a breakdown in the letterbox area, a breakdown in the phoneme-identification area, or a breakdown in the communication between the two.

There is now general consensus among researchers that the most salient problem in dyslexia is the analysis of phonemes, and that this is linked to a dysfunction of the posterior part of the midtemporal lobe (the area marked in black in Fig. 6.1).

Italian neuropsychologist Eraldo Paulesu of Milano-Bicocca University led a study of people with dyslexia from Italy, England, and France and found that irrespective of language there was an anatomical aberration and a lower degree of activity in the posterior part of the midtemporal lobe.[7],[11] Another major study compared the brain activity of seventy children with dyslexia and seventy-four children without dyslexia and found a significantly lower level of activity in both the temporal and parietal lobes.[9]

Virtually all brain imaging studies of people with dyslexia find aberrations in the same part of the brain: the posterior area of the temporal lobe (see Fig. 6.2). This said, not all scholars agree that a sound-analysis disorder is the only and definitive explanation for dyslexic problems. For example, French linguist Frank Ramus points out that a large portion of people with dyslexia seem to have problems not with phonemes but with the visual analysis of text.[13] The key question is: What is it that causes these aberrations?

DYSLEXIA: GENETICS AND DISPLACED CELLS

Dyslexia is largely inherited. However, it's a giant and difficult leap from knowing that genes matter to knowing exactly what genes they are and what function they have. Several specific genes have, however, been linked to dyslexia, in part through the research led by Swedish-Finnish geneticist Juha Keres at Karolinska Institutet. It is not yet known the precise functionality of these

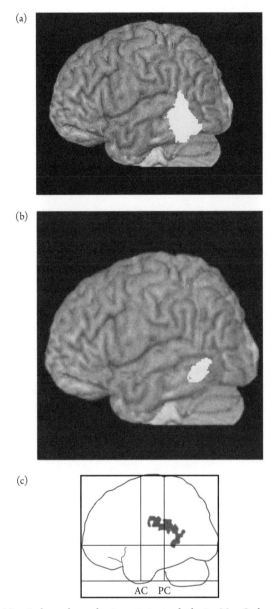

Figure 6.2 Map 1 shows lower brain activity in dyslexia. Map 2 shows changes in cortical thickness in dyslexia (from Silani, 2005).[11] Map 3 shows disruptions in the white-matter pathways (from Klingberg et al., 2000).[12]

genes, but one phenomenon that has aroused some excitement is that three of the genes (*DYX1C1*, *DCDC2*, and *KIAA0319*) have a common denominator in influencing how the cortex is formed during development.[14]

In Chapter 2 on the developing brain, it was mentioned how the cerebral cortex is formed when neurons migrate out from the center of the brain to settle in the right place in the six layers of nerve cells that comprise the roughly four millimeter thick cortex.

The hypothesis that dyslexia is related to aberrant neuronal migration also corresponds with a study from the 1980s by neurologist Albert Galaburda, who found several conglomerations of such "displaced" cells around the brains of deceased people with dyslexia, including on the temporal lobe.[15] It appeared as if the migrating cells had stopped either too early in the subcortical white matter, or too late to form small clusters of cells on the surface of the normal cortical layers. These extracellular lumps seem to corroborate the aforementioned study by Paulesu, in which people with dyslexia were found to have a characteristically thicker posterior temporal lobe than controls.

Anomalies of the nerve cells in the temporal lobe could then have knock-on effects through their influence on the development of other parts of the brain. For one thing, communication with the letterbox area should be affected, and sure enough we see lower activity in that very area. Other connections would probably be affected as well. I myself led a study in which we examined the white matter of people with dyslexia and found an aberration—most likely reduced myelination or axon thickness—in areas of white matter that lead information between the posterior language areas and the frontal lobes.[12] Our first study was of adults, but the same phenomenon has now also been observed several times in children.

There are still many unanswered questions about dyslexia. If there are genetic determinants that give rise to a dyslexogenic dysfunction in a small area at the back of the temporal lobe, there should be no connection with either dyscalculia or ADHD. But if the problem stems from neuronal migration, should this not affect the brain as a whole? Why is it just the temporal lobe?

WHY THE PROBLEMS ARE INTERCONNECTED

The simplest explanation for how problems such as dyslexia arise, namely that a genetic variation creates some sort of anomaly in

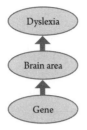

Figure 6.3 The former model of causality between genes, brain, and behavior.

the brain, is shown in Figure 6.3. This schematic model informed thinking at the end of the 1900s, but we now know that it's incorrect. A model that corresponds more closely to our current understanding is shown in Figure 6.4. The rings at the bottom of the model represent genes that code, say, for a component of a receptor, or a molecule, found on different parts of a nerve cell. The appearance and composition of the nerve cells are fairly homogenous throughout the brain. The varying thicknesses of the interconnecting lines are meant to indicate that there can be different amounts of a receptor in different areas. The "brain area" rings represent areas of roughly the same size as those shown in the maps of reading and mathematical reasoning (Fig. 6.1). The fact that they are arranged in a ring instead of a straight line illustrates the importance of their relative physical distances. These brain areas intercommunicate via pathway systems in the white matter and thus form a network able to perform certain tasks, such as keeping spatial information in working memory. This

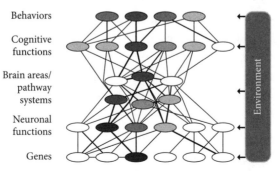

Figure 6.4 A newer model for the relationship between genes, the brain, cognitive function, and behavior.

ability, in turn, is an important aspect of a range of behaviors, such as mathematical reasoning. Diagnoses such as dyslexia, dyscalculia, and ADHD are made on the basis of behavior at the top of the network.

Much of the natural variation between individuals is more attributable to the fact that we are born with different sets of genes—the lowest level of the model. Now the reason why problems are connected is that the links between the various levels branch out. Imagine the brain regions as body parts. We all know that appearance is hereditary; you might have inherited your mother's nose or your father's stubby little toes or hair color. This is the result of common variations in our genes rather than rare mutations. It's the same with the brain. The function of different areas varies in a way that need not be judged along a unidimensional scale of better or worse, just as we don't ascribe a value to large or small feet. It's no more than natural variation of functionality.

It's rare for someone to inherit his or her father's big toe but his or her mother's little toe. Our genes often shape larger units, and it seems that this goes for the brain, too. All studies into this field of inquiry show that normal genetic variation affects regions of the brain, often several neighboring ones, that are larger than individual areas. Sometimes, such regions comprise maybe fifteen or so areas, or even the entire brain. So, for example, if you've inherited your father's dopamine receptor variant in the intraparietal cortex, it's likely that you've also inherited it in the rest of the parietal cortex, too.

We can see by looking at Figure 6.4 how one gene variation would influence the rest of the network. Imagine now that a person is defined by variations in thousands of genes. This would mean that to describe this person, one would have to superimpose a multitude of such figures. Natural variation in different brain areas and regions would then produce natural variation in psychological functions.

The fact is that natural variation in a large number of genes that affect regions of the brain tallies with most of what we know about ADHD, dyslexia, and dyscalculia. Genes that have previously been specifically linked to dyslexia also seem to show a normal variation that affects the ability to read in nondyslexic populations.[16] We mentioned that dyslexia has been associated with an aberration in the white matter (Fig. 6.2), but even in people without dyslexia there are variations in the structure of the white matter associated with differences in reading ability.[12] Instead of treating dyslexia, dyscalculia, and ADHD as "diseases" linked to a specific gene, we can see them as a manifestation of normal variation in behavior and brain function determined by a large number of genes.

DYSLEXIA TRAINING AND NEUROSCIENTIFIC PREDICTIONS

Simply because dyslexic problems are inherited and associable with specific genes and brain areas doesn't mean that we're powerless to do anything about them. Training programs designed to improve phoneme perception and letter coding allow children with dyslexia to compensate for their difficulties, even if they might never achieve real reading fluency.

Several studies have been led by American researchers Josef Torgesen and Patricia Lindamood. Swedish dyslexia researcher Ingvar Lundberg at Gothenburg University also led a productive intervention study that came to be called *The Bornholm Model*,[17] in accordance with which children receive training in analyzing and distinguishing between phonemes, in part through rhyming games. The program was conducted on six-year-olds twenty minutes a day for eight months.

Bennet Shaywitz and his colleagues at Yale University were also able to show that children who had undergone phonological training not only improved their reading, they also had a higher degree of activity in the posterior temporal lobe, the very same area that is attenuated in people with dyslexia.[18]

A practical problem with phonological training is that it's intensive and laborious. Several studies required more than fifty hours' training, spread over many months, often with a teacher who had at most three pupils. Moreover, training programs should be administered early, before children start to lag behind in their reading acquisition.

So the challenge is to find the children who need this resource-demanding training. Early tests of phonological ability can identify many children in the risk zone, but the tests are not entirely reliable. One suggestion that has attracted a degree of interest is that neuroscientists could help in the early identification of potential cases of dyslexia.

In one study led by Daniel Brandais of Zurich University, six-year-olds were studied before they started school and then given reading tests for the following five years to see which measures from the initial tests could predict future reading and writing difficulties.[19] The study included a battery of psychological tests of the children's ability to memorize and differentiate between phonemes, and electroencephalograph (EEG) readings of their brain activity. The EEG is an old tool based on measuring weak changes in potential at the scalp that occur when neurons are activated and ions flow in and out of the cells.

During the study, the researchers exposed their subjects to tones or phonemes while recording their brain activity. While they noted that the psychological tests alone were able to predict future reading and writing difficulties with some degree of reliability, they found that factoring in the EEG data significantly enhanced their predictability, enabling them to identify some eighty percent of the children who would go on to develop problems with writing and reading.

Heikki Lyytinen from the University of Jyväskylä, Finland, led a study of even younger children to find whether those in the risk zone could be identified even during infancy. The team monitored families with at least one case of dyslexia, meaning that babies in these families had about a fifty percent chance of developing it as well. On taking EEG readings of neonates as they heard phonemes such as "ba, da, ga," they found that risk-zone children displayed aberrant EEG activity even as newborn babies, unlike children outside the risk zone. It would later transpire that the EEG activity was also associated with delayed speaking skills at the ages of thirty months and five years, and reading skills at the age of six and a half.[20,21]

I began this book by asking what contributions cognitive neuroscience can make to education and our understanding of child development. The prediction of future difficulties that we've seen here is a promising area. In his article "Dyslexia: A New Strategy between Education and Cognitive Neuroscience," John Gabrieli of the Massachusetts Institute of Technology proposes that the prediction of future reading difficulties can be one of the first fields in which cognitive neuroscience will have a practical part to play, in that it can help to identify children who risk developing reading and writing difficulties so that they can be offered a proper training program in time.[22] Moreover, it's possible that reading difficulties and dyslexia are caused by dysfunctions in different brain areas, the location of which can determine the intervention to be used. The models and methods being developed for reading difficulties can then be modified to locate children who risk having difficulties in other areas.

This chapter has largely been devoted to the influence of our genes. Note, however, that unlike the older model (see Fig. 6.3), the new gene–brain area–function model contains no arrows indicating a unidirectionality of this influence; the various strata of the model can affect each other in a downward direction as well.

Phonological training is an example of how the brain can be shaped. To the right of Figure 6.4 we see the input of the environmental factor, which is something that we haven't paid much attention to yet. In the following chapters we'll therefore be taking a closer look at how environment and training influence brain structure and function, all the way down to the level of our genes.

CHAPTER 7

ᴏᐱᴏ

The Early Environment and
Brain Development

The Importance of Stimulation and
Engaged Parents

On Christmas Eve in 1989, Romanian dictator Nicolae Ceausescu was in a tank trundling along narrow roads in the west of the country—in hiding. The day before he'd addressed the crowds outside his palace, but finding his words of reassurance drowned out by the catcalls and jeers, he curtailed his command performance and fled by helicopter from the roof. The helicopter landed some miles outside Bucharest, where the dictator and his wife climbed into the waiting vehicle. Two days later they were found, still inside the tank, and hauled in front of an impromptu court. They were executed in Târgoviște village square on Christmas Day.

Ceausescu had ruled over Romania for more than two decades. On his death, many of the hidden horrors of his dictatorship were revealed to the world, such as the orphanages and the notorious regimes of maltreatment that prevailed there. These institutions were the result of Ceausescu's conscious efforts to increase the national population by fifty percent by proscribing contraceptives and abortions for women under the age of forty.

The outcome of this population control policy was involuntary large families containing sometimes six to eight children. Already bowed by the country's poor economy, many families could simply not afford to provide for all their children and turned to the only solution available: incarceration in institutions, alongside orphans and unwanted children with physical or mental disabilities.

In the early 1990s, when Romania opened its doors to the world's media, the deplorable conditions under which these institutions were run became public knowledge. An orphanage nurse sometimes had charge of as many as twenty children, all of whom received the minimal care and attention. One BBC reporter described endemic negligence and routine abuse, citing examples of children being kept in cellars for years without ever seeing the light of day.

The exposés led to widespread adoption from Romanian orphanages to the West. Many have since wondered what became of the adoptees; the Romanian orphanages constitute an extreme case study of the influence of environment on development, and it was beyond question that the children were going to be deeply affected. But would they have developed mental problems such as anxiety and depression, or impaired cognitive abilities? And was it the total time spent in the institution that was the critical factor in their possibly retarded development, or was it the age at which they were exposed to their environment?

Sensitive periods in functional development are one of the fundamental questions of developmental psychology. Some of the most seminal studies in the field were conducted in the 1960s by Swedish-American neuroscientists Torsten Wiesel and David Hubel at Harvard University, who were awarded the Nobel Prize for their contributions to science in 1981. To study how visual stimuli affect the development of the visual areas of the brain, they took newly born kittens and covered one of their eyes with a patch for three months; on removing it they found that they had induced almost total blindness in that eye, caused, it turned out, by a stunting of the interneuronal connections in the cortical areas that process visual information. When they performed the same experiment on adult cats, however, they found that their brains were not damaged in this way and that they had normal vision when the patch was removed. A lack of visual stimulation during an early, sensitive period of development was thus responsible for causing irreversible damage to the kittens' brains. A window of opportunity had been closed.

The results from Wiesel and Hubel and other studies have raised the question of whether there are similar development windows for other functions as well. Wiesel's study has often been cited to justify early schooling and cognitive training for very young children, even under the age of three. Parents' fears of missing the sensitive periods of their child's development have fuelled a flourishing industry for manufacturers of toys that allegedly stimulate everything from visual processing to cognitive skills. Many scholars, myself included, refute the validity of these interpretations. First, the studies demonstrated that a total absence of stimulation affected brain architecture, not that increased stimulation benefited powers of vision any more than the visual input that kittens normally receive. Second, subsequent research suggests that the concept of a window that is either open or closed is a rather simplified one. Animals that are stimulus-deprived for a shorter period of time when young can partly recover their visual functionality if they then receive normal stimulation. So rather than being black and white, the window is shaded in nuances of gray. Third, sensitive periods have been mainly documented in the development of *sensory* systems. We know that foreign languages are best learned before the age of ten to twelve if they're to be spoken without a mother-tongue accent, which is an example of a kind of sensitive period of language development, but this too is a gray zone, and adults can also learn to speak new languages. As for *cognitive* development, however, the subject of sensitivity in humans is still very much terra incognita.

British child psychiatrist Michael Rutter took an early interest in "Ceausescu's orphans" and has published a number of papers comparing the development of children adopted from Romanian institutions into UK homes with Romanian adoptees without an institutional background and children adopted within the United Kingdom.[1],[2]

The picture that has emerged is a depressing one. All the Romanian children in Rutter's studies were adopted before the age of three and a half. When they were examined at the age of eleven, the group as a whole had significantly lower attainments scores in almost every field measured, the lowest being registered by those who had been adopted after the age of six months. The children from Romanian institutions performed worse on tests of both reading and mathematics, and general IQ tests indicated an impairment of roughly twenty points compared with the group of children adopted from within the United Kingdom, placing them all among the ten to fifteen percent poorest performers.

When Rutter and colleagues examined the children, they found that sixty-six percent of them had some form of psychiatric symptom, as opposed to twenty percent of the control group. They displayed autistic symptoms with impaired social interaction, emotional dysfunction, attention disorders, and hyperactivity. As regards the time of adoption, the most striking observation was that those who were adopted before the age of six months fared much better than those adopted later, suggesting six months as a possible starting point for our conjectural sensitive period.

One methodological problem with Rutter's studies is that it's hard to tell what caused the children to be placed in the orphanage in the first place. The group adopted before the age of six months also manifested certain problems, but it's difficult to determine the extent to which they postdated or predated their institutionalization. A strictly scientific study of environmental effects would have to be randomized and controlled, and involve comparing the development of two groups of children from an orphanage, one having been blindly assigned to foster parents.

One such randomized study of children from Romanian institutions was conducted by a group of researchers from the United States led by Charles Nelson III from Harvard Medical School. It might seem unethical to manipulate the destinies of children for the sake of science like this, and indeed the study has not been without its detractors. In their defence, however, the researchers pointed out that when the study began there was no adoption system in place within Romania, so if it hadn't been for their research grant, most of the children would probably have been left to the mercy of the institutions.

Their initial study was published in *Science* in 2007.[3] To measure the effects of environment, the team focused on cognitive development measured using a battery of IQ tests when the children were four and a half years old. Their first conclusion was that adoption benefited cognition, as the adopted children performed on average eight percent better on IQ tests than their peers in the orphanages, the best scores being attained by those who had been adopted before the age of two. Adoption had a positive impact on all age groups, so the boundaries were not absolute; but if the adoptions took place before the children had reached the age of two, the effect was almost double that seen in those adopted later, a finding that substantiates, in part at least, the theories of developmental sensitivity.

Although impoverished environment will always undermine the maturation of the growing brain, cognitive development seems to be extremely environmentally sensitive between the ages of six months and two years. It should be pointed out, however, that these orphanage studies are extreme and need carry no wider social implications. Moreover, there are two components of the children's environment that could have impacted on their development: lack of parental interaction and understimulation.

STIMULATING ENVIRONMENTS AND BRAIN DEVELOPMENT

New parents tend to find their letterboxes overflowing with advertising material from companies keen to exploit their eagerness to give their offspring the very best and most secure childhoods, complete with the safest toys, the driest diapers, and the utmost stimulation. Diaper dryness can be measured; optimal stimulation, on the other hand, is hard to gauge.

The effects of stimulating, or enriching, environments have been studied in animals since the 1940s. It was back then that

Canadian psychologist Donald Hebb first reported on enriched environments for rats. While conducting his experiments on the rodent memory, he would sometimes take some of his rats home for his children to play with. To his surprise, he found that the rats that had been allowed to run freely around his house subsequently performed better on the memory tasks he put them through in his laboratory. In the decades since, scientists have been studying the effects of "enrichment" by transferring their experimental mice or rats from the traditional barren plastic cages in which laboratory animals are normally kept to larger, more populated cages containing tunnels, steps, exercise wheels, and objects for the animals to explore. These environments give them more opportunities for interaction, both with their surroundings and with other animals. Animals kept in such spaces subsequently perform better on memory tasks, such as solving mazes (see Fig. 7.1).[4]

No single factor has yet been identified to explain the full effect of enriched environments. Just letting a rat observe a stimulating environment through a glass window without letting it integrate with it (what they call a "TV rat") produces no improvement in memory. The social stimulation obtained by having several rats occupy the same cage has a certain effect, but not as much as when the cage is also full of toys. The physical activity that the enriched environment provides seems to have an effect in and of itself, and simply introducing an exercise wheel for a rat to run

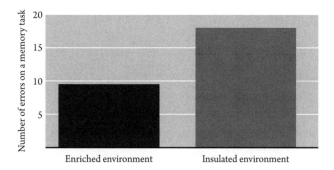

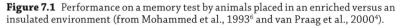

Figure 7.1 Performance on a memory test by animals placed in an enriched versus an insulated environment (from Mohammed et al., 1993[6] and van Praag et al., 2000[4]).

around in (the "gym rat") improves the memory, a phenomenon I will be describing later in Chapter 10. Nevertheless, this single phenomenon cannot explain the overall effects of the enriched environment as a whole.

There are several changes in brain morphology in animals from enriched environments. William Greenough from the University of Illinois has conducted several important studies in this field, and concluded at the end of one review paper covering decades of research on stimulation and the brain, seemingly quite overwhelmed by the sheer volume of data and results, that "the most general conclusion that can be made confidently is that the brain is an extremely plastic organ."[5]

Some specific findings, however, are worth discussing. One distinct change in brain architecture is that enriched environments increase the number and length of dendrites and the number of synapses on each neuron; they also stimulate the proliferation of neurons in the hippocampus, or more accurately the gyrus dentatus, the part of the hippocampus in which the formation of new nerve cells occurs, a phenomenon that we have seen is associated with the long-term memory. It's impossible that a single factor underlies both synapse propagation and neuron formation, and there are many chemical candidates for these effects. One is a growth hormone called the Brain-Derived Neurotrophic Factor (BDNF), higher concentrations of which are found in the hippocampuses of rats from enriched environments. One difference between the studies of visual development in cats (e.g., Hubel and Wiesel) and of enriched environments in rats is that in the latter case the positive effects of stimulation are also found in adults—which might offer you a crumb of comfort if you think your office cubicle more resembles a bare, toyless rat cage; it's never too late to change.

Like Wiesel's study, the research on stimulating environments is often cited by advocates of early schooling or of the optimal stimulation of three-year-olds. I myself suspect that the rats' enriched environment is more like the normal habitat of a wild rat. If this is so, the results should be interpreted as the effect not of stimulation but of negligence contra a normal upbringing. It is thus more like a parallel to the impairments observed in the children from the Romanian orphanages, not what can be expected of children placed in hyperstimulating preschools. The effects of the early childhood environment are analogous to those of some vitamins: a lack of vitamin C leads to scurvy, but taking three times the recommended daily dose has no extra benefits as the surplus is merely excreted in the urine. In fact, some vitamins can even be harmful in excess amounts. The validity of this analogy remains an open question; and even if it did hold, we would still have no idea what the recommended daily dose of stimulation would be.

One set of results that support the notion of a parallel between enriched and natural environments come from a study on brain cell formation in wild birds.[7] After injecting a substance into trapped birds that would enable them to detect the number of new cells formed, they released some of the birds into the wild and kept the remainder in captivity. On subsequently retrapping some of the tagged "wild" population they found that they had a larger proportion of newly formed nerve cells in the part of the brain corresponding to the hippocampus, just like the rats from the enriched environments. This leads us to conclude that the natural habitat is more like the artificial enriched environment than it is the bare, sterile one. Wild birds apparently don't only have the most beautiful songs; they also have the more stimulated brains.

THE ROLE OF PARENTS IN MEMORY AND STRESS

A lack of stimulation is one of the possible detriments to development in the Romanian orphanages. Another is the lack of parental contact. The importance of parental bonding has been a topic of much study in the psychology of attachment, and in animal studies of the infant environment, it has also been possible to see the effects of parenting on cerebral development. Mother rats, for example, suckle their offspring for their first weeks of life, during which time she also fusses over them by licking them and providing plenty of physical contact. However, there is natural variation in how attentive mother rats are (something that has been particularly studied in the common brown rat, *rattus norvegicus*).

Neuroscientist Michael Meaney at McGill University in Canada sought to find out the effects that maternal caregiving had on development. By observing how much time mother rats spent licking their young, he and his team identified a group of infants with extremely caring mothers and a group with mothers that were more negligent and that licked their offspring half as frequently. The infant rats were subsequently tested for long-term memory once they had matured. Meaney found that the rats raised by the caring mothers had a better learning capacity than those from the negligent group,[8] and that this cognitive improvement was associated with a higher population of synapses in the hippocampus. They also noted higher concentrations of the growth factor BDNF and of NMDA receptors, which are important to the encoding of long-term memories. Maternal caregiving during the first ten days of life thus permanently influenced the young rats' learning abilities.

For the second part of their study, Meaney's team gave the experiment an interesting tweak. They knew which mother rats were the more or less attentive, and that their caring patterns were repeated for every litter they bore. So the researchers conducted a little adopting experiment, and when the mother rats next produced new litters they swapped some of the young from the negligent mothers with an equal number of young from the caring mothers. They subsequently found that the young that had been adopted by the caring mothers performed just as well on memory tasks as her own biological infants and had the corresponding increase in synapses, BDNF, and NMDA receptors.

The attentiveness of rat mothers not only affects their infants' memories but also their stress tolerance. One method of measuring stress reactions is to place a rat in a new, circular cage that has a wall but no corners in which to seek shelter. Open spaces are frightening to rats, but they're also inquisitive and exploratory, which means that rats with a lower stress overload will spend more time in the open, while their more neurotic peers will tend to prowl around the edge of the cage. Meaney and his team showed that caring mother rats have young that grow up to become less easily stressed and more likely to spend time in the open in new cages (see Fig. 7.2).[9] The better stress tolerance is also linked to differences in the number of brain receptors for the stress hormone cortisol. Furthermore, young rats adopted from a negligent mother by a caring mother and vice versa are affected by the adoptive mother's behavior rather than that of their biological mother, so the offspring of a negligent mother transferred to a caring mother show just as much stress tolerance as the caring mother's own biological litter.

The effects of adoption are indeed fascinating in themselves, but Meaney took a step further and examined how the adopted female young themselves behaved when they had their own litters. It turned out that the young of negligent mothers adopted by caring mothers not only displayed higher stress tolerance but also became caring mothers that had stress-tolerant litters. The results illustrate how acquired characteristics can be inherited.

When I was a medical student in the 1990s, such Lamarckian inheritance was still totally implausible. Characteristics were

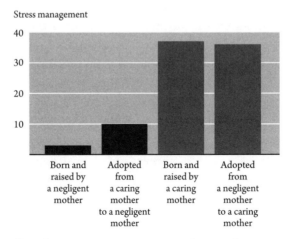

Figure 7.2 Effect of caring on stress management (measured as time spent in open spaces).[9]

passed on from generation to generation exclusively via the genes, and it was just a handful of politically motivated Soviet scientists who claimed that acquired characteristics could be inherited. The explanation, it would transpire, is that genes can be modified, and how this happens is now a hot research field called *epigenetics*.

Genes consist of DNA molecules that specify how a specific protein is to be manufactured. Experiences cannot change our DNA; they *can*, however, affect how much of the protein is to be synthesized, which is exactly what Michael Meaney has shown happens in the offspring of the caring mother rats. Through the agency of a biochemical reaction called methylation which takes place during the first eight days of life, a modification occurs in their DNA that permanently changes the number of stress hormone receptors expressed.[10]

In the United States, over 3.3 million cases of child abuse are reported every year; just how many cases there are that don't get reported is anyone's guess. A traumatic childhood is a primary cause of anxiety, depression, and suicidal tendencies later in life. To study whether the biochemical mechanisms they had observed in animals applied to children, Meaney and his team examined the brains of twelve adult suicide victims who had also been the victims of childhood abuse, and compared them with those of suicide victims who had not been abused as children and of people who had died of other causes than suicide.[11] In those that had been subjected to abuse, they found the same change in expression of the stress hormone receptor as they had observed in the offspring of the negligent mother rats, and could attribute the difference in receptor population to the methylation of their DNA. Early experiences thus produce biochemical changes in the brain and genes that are of the utmost relevance.

The Romanian children have met different destinies: some live on the street; others live well-ordered lives with jobs and families. Some returned to the institutions as workers to give their charges a better upbringing than they themselves had; others just try to forget. When BBC reporter Kate McGeown visited

Romania in 2005 to find out what became of the children, she recognized a young man whom she'd last seen as a child in one of the orphanages. She asked him to tell her of his experiences of growing up there: "I would love to help you," he said. "But I wasn't there."

CHAPTER 8

cⱱɔ

Skydiving and Expectations

What Acute and Chronic Stress Do to Us

In 2004, a thirty-something man died after his parachute failed to open. When his equipment was examined, it was found he'd never even tried to release his reserve parachute, which was intact and fully functional. The interpretation was that the jumper had suffered a stress overload that had given him such a mental block that he couldn't remember what to do or think clearly enough to take the right action. A study of skydiving fatalities in the United States in the 1990s classified eleven percent as "no pull."[1] A fatal consequence of stress.

An individual's cognitive abilities are partly inherited but remain nonetheless far from constant. In Chapter 7 we saw how childhood experiences can form the brain and affect cognitive function. There are also more fast-acting effects that change a person's abilities from one day to another, even from minute to minute. One of the most significant factors behind such effects turns out to be stress.

Psychologists John Leach and Rebecca Griffith at Lancaster University in the United Kingdom decided to look into how stress caused by skydiving influences working memory.[2] While one accompanied the skydivers in the plane and tested their working memory during the minutes before they were due to jump, the other waited at the landing site to test their working memory the moment they landed. They also tested each jumper in a stress-free control environment. What they found was that their prejump stress seriously impaired their working memory. Even experienced skydivers with over forty jumps under their belts performed thirty percent worse on the memory test than they did in the calm of the control situation; beginners had as much as a forty percent impairment. When the experienced sky-divers were tested on landing, they performed on par with their normal level; the beginners, on the other hand, were apparently still more or less terrified on reaching terra firma, their working memory performance rising merely to thirty percent below nor-mal. Granted, it might not be that surprising to find that people aren't at their cognitive bests just before they're due to jump out of an airplane at an altitude of 2,000 meters (or roughly 6,500 feet), but the magnitude of the impairment is remarkable. Acute stress can almost halve a person's mental capacity.

Now I've never skydived, and life in the lab is hardly life-threatening. Giving a lecture is pretty much the most stressful thing I experience on a daily basis. But even though I've given hundreds of lectures, my pulse still starts to race and my brow to bead with sweat as I climb onto the stage whether it be to fifty or five hundred eyes staring at me. Luckily, I've learned to over-come the stress and, just like the experienced skydivers, manage to recover my normal working memory capacity and land rela-tively unscathed.

I'm not the only one to find lecturing stressful. Stress overload on giving a presentation to a group is such a general and relia-ble reaction that it's often used as an experimental method for studying the effects of stress. One version of lecture stress is called the *Trier Social Stress Test*, in which participants are asked to deliver a five-minute talk to an audience of psychologists who will be recording, judging, and critiquing their performance. In one study that measured the physiological reactions of such subjects, researchers observed elevated blood levels of the stress hormone cortisol and an increase in pulse and blood pressure.[3] They also found that raised cortisol levels undermined working memory. The effects were not as dramatic as for the skydivers, but the lecture situation still resulted in a ten percent drop in performance.

The effects of stress are probably pertinent to school children, too. Töres Theorell from Karolinska Institutet along with Mats Lundahl and Frank Lindblad from Linneaus University in Kalmar studied a group of seventh and ninth graders as they did math tests, and measured their cortisol levels.[4] They found that children with a high level of stress had more cortisol in their blood, hyperventilated more, and underperformed compared with their low-cortisol peers. A higher stress reaction was also linked to lower self-confidence. So let's take a closer look at what happens during a stress reaction and how it might explain the changes we observe in working and long-term memory.

STRESS HORMONES AND NERVE CELLS

The stress reaction prepares the body for "flight or fight." Blood is channelled into the muscles while the skin capillaries contract, the pupils dilate, and the sweat glands open, rendering the stressed person looking pale and in a cold sweat. Noradrenalin (norepinephrine) is one of the key stress-related neurotransmitters in the brain and is also what makes us extra alert when something interesting or unexpected happens nearby. In fact, the difference between being drowsy, alert, or stressed is largely just a matter of noradrenalin concentrations.

Noradrenalin attaches itself to receptors that can be found in most parts of the brain, not least of all the prefrontal cortex. It also stimulates the amygdala (the deep-lying cell group that we discussed in Chapter 3). If the hippocampus is the seat of the memory, then the amygdala can be thought of as the seat of fear.

When we're stressed, our bodies also secrete adrenalin and cortisol into the blood, which affects almost every body organ. Adrenalin is blocked by the blood-brain barrier but not cortisol, which floods into the brain attaching itself to the relatively ubiquitous glucocorticoid receptor. There is a particular concentration of these receptors in the amygdala and hippocampus, and this affects both our stress reaction and memory. Activation of the glucocorticoid receptors creates a negative feedback loop, which reduces the stress reaction like a built-in brake that restores balance to the system. The lion that frightens the zebra activates the zebra's stress reaction, which prepares it for flight; but once the lion's out of sight, this negative feedback loop brings the zebra's system back to its normal state of balance so that it can go on grazing.

The offspring of the mother rats we met in Chapter 7 had a lower concentration of glucocorticoid receptors in the hippocampus, which undermined hippocampal function and the encoding of long-term memories. It also resulted in a poorer system brake, an exaggerated stress reaction, and neurotic rats that even as adults would skulk along the edges of their cages.

Stress has a complex effect on the memory that depends not only on the degree of stress but also on the type of memory, as the long-term and working memories are affected differently. And then there's chronic stress, which is another phenomenon altogether.

At times of acute stress, cortisol, noradrenalin, and amygdala activation actually improve long-term memory encoding,[5] hence the so-called flashbulb memories that allow us to remember emotional situations, such as accidents, with particular clarity. Most of us can say where we were when we heard the news of 9/11 or the Asian tsunami. Many fewer would be able to say what they were doing the day before. In evolutionary terms, it's logical for us to imprint dangerous situations—such as that tree where that lion last appeared—with extra clarity so that we may avoid them in the future. But stimuli don't have to be as serious as disasters or life-threatening situations for the amygdala to boost our memory. All it takes is for a text to include a description of an accident for us to remember it better than we do a text describing a walk in the park. We also code faces depicting anxiety or anger better than we do those with neutral expressions. Generally speaking, experiences and information that carry some kind of emotional association create more lasting memories.

Working memory, however, improves at a fair degree of alertness but deteriorates at times of high stress. This is usually described as an inverted-U function. There is an optimal level of stress, and either too much or too little undermines performance. Again, the culprits are cortisol and noradrenalin. We can show that the firing of individual neurons in the prefrontal cortex also obey an inverted-U function, with the peak occurring at the optimal level of noradrenalin.[6] Even though a person's performance is not determined by a certain neuron, we still see the same inverted-U pattern at both the lowest neuronal level and the highest behavioral level, in much the same way as we see fractal forms in the macro and the microworlds.

Unlike the encoding of long-term memories, their retrieval is debilitated by acute stress.[5] Memory retrieval requires the activation of the prefrontal cortex, a phenomenon that could be explained by the same function as for working memory—and one that is all too familiar to anyone who's been under time pressure during an exam and with heart racing and armpits sweating has totally failed to summon up the smallest nugget of relevant information.

SOCIAL STRESS

Humans are social beings, for good or ill. Social contacts can be our most valuable asset, but other people, to paraphrase Sartre, can be hell. The stress we feel during a lecture is an example of social stress. Other people's expectations, or rather what we imagine their expectations to be, can also cause us stress. The scientific name for this kind of stress is *stereotype threat*.

Two of the first psychologists to demonstrate this effect were Claude Steele and Joshua Aronson of Stanford University,[7] who sought to study the differences in IQ test performance between Afro-American and Caucasian students that had been documented by several previous studies. Their hypothesis was that the awareness of the general conception that Black people underperform White people on intelligence tests gave rise to a fear in the former to confirm the stereotype, which undermines their performance. They were able to show that the performance of their Black subjects, but not the White, was affected by whether the test was presented as an evaluation of racial differences. When it was

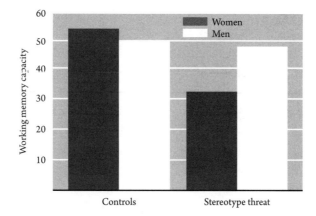

Figure 8.1 Effect of stress on working memory caused by "stereotype threat" in men and women (from Schmader and Johns, 2003).[8]

presented in neutral terms that had no direct association with racial prejudice, the groups performed equally well. Their results have since been corroborated by studies of other minority groups.

Toni Schmader and Michael Johns from the University of Arizona wanted to examine whether the stereotype threat could also influence women's performance on a test of mathematics (see Fig. 8.1).[8] So they had their male and female subjects answer a number of mathematical statements and remember a word that followed each one.

Example:
(3 x 2) – 1 = 4   yes/no   Apple
(12/3) + 1 = 5   yes/no   Sofa

Here, the subjects would have to answer no, remember the word "apple", answer yes, remember the word "sofa", and hten recall the memorised words "apple, sofa".

This is a very common psychological test, but one that is normally used to measure working memory capacity rather than mathematical skills.

The subjects were divided into two groups, the first a control group who were told that they were to carry out a test of their working memory, the other an experimental group who were told that the researchers wanted to evaluate their "quantitative capacity"—the ability to solve complex mathematical problems while holding nonmathematical information in the memory. This group were also asked to indicate their sex on the test paper before commencing as differences in performance could depend on gender differences in "quantitative capacity."

Both groups performed identical tasks. In the control group, men and women performed fairly equally. However, when the test was presented as a math test that was potentially susceptible to possible gender influences, the men's performance was largely unaffected while the women's performance deteriorated by forty percent compared to the controls.

Their next experiment involved just women, who performed a verbal working memory test and a mathematical task. The control group were told that they were to perform a memory test and reasoning test in order to provide the researchers with a mean value for normal college student performance. The experimental group, who were to be subjected to stereotype threat, were told that they were to perform a mathematical test so that the researchers could compare gender differences in mathematical skills.

The control group was only women; the "threat" group, however, took the test in groups of two men and one woman. They found that the woman in the "threat" group performed worse not only on the working memory test but also thirty percent worse than the women in the control group on the math task. The deterioration of working memory could explain their impaired performance on the math test; that is to say that if the researchers statistically removed every discrepancy in mathematical score that could be attributed to differences in working memory, then the differences in mathematical performance between the groups would also disappear. It thus seemed that expectations created stress and stress debilitated working memory, which in turn undermined mathematical performance.

In Chapter 5 we saw that the gap between girls and boys in terms of mathematical skills has gradually narrowed over the years and that gender differences in this respect correlate with equality in the rest of society. However, just how such a correlation could arise was unclear. Schmader and John's results provide a possible causal explanation. In the countries where boys perform better than girls, the difference is only one or two percent. The effect of negative expectations can drag performance down by up to thirty percent and might well explain the gender differences seen between countries. Stress research also gives us the biological mechanisms: the debilitation of working memory due to an excess of cortisol and noradrenalin.

CHRONIC STRESS

When the lion is out of sight, the built-in braking mechanism restores balance to the zebra's stress system. If this balance is not restored and the stress overload continues, it's called chronic stress and produces an array of negative effects. Human beings, with their complex social environment and ability to plan for the future, are particularly susceptible to the phenomenon. Zebras simply don't have the same tendency to lie in their beds sleepless at night worrying about their mortgages.

The stress overload caused by skydiving, lecturing, and stereotype threat is an acute reaction that peters out within the space of an hour. But if the stress becomes chronic and the brain has no chance to recover, changes take place to nerve cells and receptors that reduce functionality and that alter how the stress system responds to new stressful situations. One theory is that neurons in the amygdala are modulated to increase the number of activating synapses, while the signals that are meant to mitigate the stress reaction decrease. The amygdala thus becomes hyperactive, leading to pathological anxiety.[5]

Chronic stress has several marked effects on the brain, including a retardation of new nerve cell production in the hippocampus, and a contraction of the projections on the neurons already there. The projections also become stunted in the prefrontal cortex by as much as thirty percent.[6] The cortex literally shrinks. Fortunately these architectural changes are reversible. In mice

exposed to twenty days of stress, nerve cells return to their normal size after three weeks without stress.[9]

In students, who in one study were subjected to stress in the
form of four weeks' preparations for an important exam, the correlation of activity in the frontal lobes with other areas of the
brain was observed to deteriorate.[10] This could be the result of
dendrite shrinkage that has been seen in mice after exposure to
chronic stress. Dendrites are the projections that receive signals
from other parts of the brain, and their shrinkage would prejudice communication with other cortical neurons, which under
the magnetic resonance scanner is seen as a reduced correlation
between brain areas. When the stressed students were allowed
to rest for four weeks, their performance and their brain activity
were fortunately restored.

The effects of chronic stress have been predominantly studied
in animals and adult humans, but its prevalence among children
and the effect it has on them are less well documented. As we have
seen, the caring behavior of mothers during infancy shapes children's stress tolerance as adults, and one circumstance that could
contribute to chronic social stress is being raised in an impoverished environment. In one American study, 196 children, half of
whom spent most or all of their childhood in homes falling below
the official US poverty line, were monitored over a period of several years.[11] Indirect measurements of chronic stress, such as
blood pressure, body mass index, cortisol and noradrenalin, were
taken at the ages of nine and thirteen and then aggregated into
a single physiological stress rating. At the age of seventeen, the
subjects' working memories were tested and an estimate made of
the percentage of their childhood spent in impoverished circumstances. The first analysis showed that children from poor families had lower working memories than their middle-class peers,
and that this impairment correlated with the proportion of their
childhood that was spent in poverty.

What the researchers then observed was that the physiological stress rating could explain the connection between poverty
and working memory, and when they statistically controlled
for differences in stress, the relationship duly disappeared. The

mechanisms behind this phenomenon could be the same as those found in mice or students, where prolonged stress overload caused observable cortical damage. On briefer exposure to stress, a shorter period of recovery is sufficient; how recovery takes place after a stressed childhood is harder to say.

What is the most critical determinant of stress in middle-class children? Stress is often correlated with other psychiatric symptoms, such as depression. In a review paper from the Royal Swedish Academy of Sciences, it was established that mental health and school performance are mutually influential, in that poor mental health affects performance, and vice versa.[12] The report also cites a similar paper written by Erica Frydenberg from the University of Melbourne in 2008, which defines three stress-inducing factors in teenagers: (1) school performance, (2) friends and family, and (3) social circumstances, including poverty. This means that poor early performance at school can lead a child into a descending spiral of failure and stress.

Fears are often voiced that the increasing swell of information in the burgeoning information technology society, with its demand for permanent Internet connections, unemptied e-mail inboxes, Facebook, Twitter, and games, could lead to a general rise in stress levels. In my book *The Overflowing Brain*, I tried to give an account of the known correlational phenomena. Playing computer games, for instance, doesn't impair attention or working memory. We must also distinguish between handling a heavy information load on the one hand and feeling anxiety and stress on the other. A long-term care worker can become burned out by constant worry while a CEO of a multibillion company might not, despite her handling much more information. What matters is more a question of how we react to our environment. A constant torrent of text messages might give you stress overload, but for your teenage daughter it might be a sign of a healthy social life that actually lowers her levels of stress.

Since stress is an important influencer of cognitive function, especially working memory, greater pains should be taken to root out the causes of stress. That poverty is a cause of chronic stress and impaired working memory has an obvious implication: we must fight poverty. But how to do this is no simple matter. The vicious circle of school performance and stress should be broken through early intervention for risk zone children, and our understanding of how prejudice and stereotype threat affect performance could certainly be put to constructive use. Indeed, most of the researchers behind these studies also believe that since the effect is a subtle one and only exists by virtue of the situation and the individual's own attitude, it could be eradicated simply by exposing the mechanisms at play.

Whatever the causes of stress, there's an abundance of methods for counteracting its symptoms. Relaxation, yoga, mindfulness training, and meditation have been studied in adults and have shown to be of possible benefit in their temporary easing of stress; several studies are currently under way to find out whether similar activities can help children. And as we'll see later, exercise also seems to be an effective way to reduce stress.

And finally: if you ever feel the urge to go skydiving, I suggest you make sure to use a reserve parachute that opens automatically.

CHAPTER 9

༄

Cognitive Training, Memory Techniques, and Music

The studies of the Romanian children's homes show just how detrimental an impoverished environment can be to development. But is there anything that could have a positive effect, over and above the ingredients of a relatively normal upbringing, such as social contacts, caring parents, toys, books, and a decent school? More specifically: Can cognitive functions be enhanced?

To evaluate the effects of "brain training," in 2009 the BBC embarked on a study of 14,000 participants.[1] The subjects were divided into three groups: two would perform tasks that could vaguely be labeled "brain training" with diverse kinds of memory and reasoning exercises, while the control group would do a form of quiz. The participants were asked to do the various tests online twice a week for six weeks. This was to be the largest training study ever conducted; but the fact that it ever even got off the ground is in itself remarkable. Hadn't research come any further than this by 2009? Don't we know whether cognitive functions can be trained?

Despite the volumes of evidence we have on how the brain is shaped by experience and training, the question of memory training, powers of concentration, and reasoning is still frustratingly contradictory. To sort out the concepts, we should first distinguish between the training of specific strategies and techniques, and the training of general skills. If we were to draw a comparison with physical training, the learning of specific techniques would equate to how you learn to deliver a decent serve on the tennis court or angle your skies properly to negotiate the gates on a slalom course. Such strategy training will improve your skills, but you will see no spreading effect whereby your more accurate serves will make you a more accomplished skier. General ability training can be likened to going to the gym and building up a particular muscle group or improving your cardiovascular fitness; stronger legs or a better oxygen uptake will probably benefit your tennis and your skiing. In cognitive terms, an example of strategy training is the techniques people use for memorizing lists of words or numbers; examples of general training, as described later in the chapter, are the training of working memory and the effect of playing a musical instrument.

THE DREAM OF THE PERFECT MEMORY

In 2010, Ben Pridmore, a thirty-something accountant from Derby in the United Kingdom, won the World Memory Championships, which since 1991 have been held to celebrate the art of memorization, with such exciting events as memorizing as many ones and zeros from a list as possible in thirty minutes, memorizing names and faces in fifteen minutes, or memorizing the order of cards in a deck. Ben holds the world record in many such events and can memorize the cards in a deck in twenty-five seconds. In an hour he can memorize twenty-five different packs and can learn 4,140 random digits in half an hour.

How does he do it? Unlike many other contestants, Ben is generous with his tricks, which he refers to as "Ben's system." To remember numbers, he has linked every three-digit combination to a specific object or person, so that 102 might be Don Draper (from the TV series *Mad Men*), 839 a combine-harvester, and 564 a billiard ball. These images can then be combined into a composite image: Don Draper driving a combine-harvester through a sea of billiard balls, which represents the sequence 102839564. Such images are then strung together into a kind of storyboard that runs around the walls of a familiar building, which in Ben's own case are the classrooms and corridors of his old school. To remember the playing cards, he has an image for each pairing of cards: the queen of diamonds and the two of spades being represented by a teacup, for example. So if you want to be as good at remembering cards as Ben, all you have to do is create a system of 2,652 images representing all possible permutations of two cards. But I suppose you might have better things to occupy your time.

To make memorizing this enormous library of images easier, Ben also has a system of translating numbers into sounds. If the first digit of a three-digit number is 1, the word will start with "d," the second digit 0 gives "o," and the third digit 2 gives "n": the word for the number 102 will therefore begin with "don."

The strategies that Ben Pridmore uses are variations of common mnemonic techniques, strategies that were described back in ancient times by classical Greeks and Romans. The first story of the mnemonic technique is usually ascribed to Simonides from Ceos. He was once attending a party, and while he happened to be outside the house, the roof suddenly caved in. Afterward he was able to recite the names of all the guests by associating them to where they were sitting at the table. The Romans developed the technique by devising the memory palace to remember different parts of a long speech they were to hold in the senate. Different parts of the speech were associated with objects placed around the palace or in the room in which they were due to perform. When it was then time to hold the speech, they'd do so by mentally walking around their memory palace. Such associations are a version of the "levels of processing" idea, which shows that we remember something better if we link it to previously stored knowledge.

Association techniques might find their use for certain school tasks, such as learning the vocabulary of a foreign language. Special pedagogue Margo Mastropieri and Thomas Scruggs of the University of Purdue in Indiana have given some concrete advice on how to use these methods for learning in school. To remember that *phanerogames* means flowering plants, the new word is associated with a picture the sound of which recalls the word, in this case "fan" maybe. The image of a fan is then paired with one of the flowers, ideally in a slightly absurd way, maybe a flower with its petals blown back by the draught of a big Japanese fan. Numerical information is memorized in a similar way to that described by Ben Pridmore, by building up a library of standard associations between digits and words: one—bun, two—shoe, three—tree, four—floor, five—hive, six—sticks, and so forth.

To remember that insects have six legs, one might think of a huge insect sculpture made of sticks. Several studies by Mastropieri and Scruggs have also shown that this is particularly useful in schools for children with learning difficulties.[2],[3]

THE BRAIN OF A MEMORY CHAMPION

Memorizing a six-digit telephone number is a relatively difficult thing to do. But isn't there something special about the brain of the memory champion who's able to learn 4,140 numbers in half an hour? Eleanor Maguire, cognitive neuroscientist at London's University College, studied ten of the contenders in the World Memory Championship who had trained memory techniques for an average of eleven years, and compared them with ten controls with a normal memory.[4] First, she let the participants perform some tests designed to measure reasoning skills, such as finding patterns in matrices of symbols and drawing inferences from them. Here, the groups performed equally well. Next, she had them carry out a memory task in which they had to copy a picture composed of geometric figures, once when the picture was still visible and again thirty minutes later from memory. Surprisingly, this was a task that the memory champions didn't particularly excel at either, there being no significant difference between their performance and that of the controls. When the participants were required to remember numbers, however, the memory champions were far superior.

It seems, then, that the memory champions' strategies worked only for a certain type of information, for when they were presented with an entirely novel problem for which they were unable to apply their mnemonic strategy, they proved to have perfectly normal memory skills. Ben Pridmore also describes how he's forever forgetting his friends' birthdays, and other memory champions talk of how they'd be unable to manage without post-it notes reminding them to do everything from make a phone call to take their wallet with them when they go to work in the morning.

So a memory champion apparently has no generally superior ability to establish synapses or an especially productive hippocampus, as is confirmed by the work of Eleanor Maguire, whose inquiries into the phenomenon found no differences between the brain structures of memory champions and controls.

The results of this study show that memory champions do not have advanced intellects or special brains. Nor does it seem as if their hippocampuses had been altered by years of memorizing. They're excellent at remembering things, but only if it's information that allows them to use their learned association methods. In other words, you or I would be just as good at learning these strategies. One anecdote that seems to confirm this is told by journalist Joshua Foer, who was asked by the magazine *Slate* to report from one of these memory championships. He became fascinated by the phenomenon and decided to learn the association techniques himself, which he recorded in his book *Moonwalking with Einstein*. After a year's training Foer went on to win the US memory championship. But the training didn't seem to have affected his normal life to any significant extent. As he put it himself in a radio interview: "I'm the person who, you know, shampoos his hair twice in the morning because he forgot that he had just done it."

Back in Chapter 5 we met Daniel Tammet, who has an exceptional ability not only to calculate but also to remember strings of digits, such as the 22,514 decimals of pi. In Daniel's case, too, it's the association of images and numbers that enables him to perform such feats of memory. Daniel argues in his autobiography that he was born with an automatic associative ability that gives the exceptional ability with numbers, while the likes of Ben, the accountant, have to learn them consciously.

Joshua Foer has met Daniel Tammet on several occasions, and every time has been struck by how his prodigious numerical memory isn't that unusual compared with the feats that other memory champions, including Joshua himself, can perform with the aid of mnemonic techniques and diligent practice. Even Daniel's other abilities, such as the mental multiplication of multidigit numbers, can be trained using well-known techniques. So the question is whether Daniel really does have a unique innate ability, or whether he's just a generally gifted person who has learned memorization techniques and passed himself off as a savant. Foer also shows convincingly that Daniel has withheld information on how much training he has actually done using memorization techniques.

The fact remains, however, that Daniel has been examined by experts in the field of synaesthesia, including Simon Barron-Cohen, who have concluded that his is a case of distinct synaesthesia. Foer's objection is that everyone who's trained his or her memory using mnemonic techniques that entail the perpetual association of images and numbers would pass Barron-Cohen's synaesthesia tests. And if we look again at the results of Daniel Tammet's magnetic resonance (MR) scan, we actually see none of the visual area activity that we might expect.

As a final test of Daniel's alleged ability to produce images for different numbers, Joshua asked him on three separate occasions about the image conjured up by the number 9412. He received a different answer each time.

The images that Daniel Tammet visualizes are known only to himself. But it seems likely that his numerical skills are not innate but the outcome of specific mnemonic techniques and a lot of practice. Rather than being unique, his abilities are something that Joshua Foer, you, and I could learn. Which is in itself a positive message to take away.

WORKING MEMORY TRAINING

For decades, psychologists have portrayed working memory as a box: a container of fixed dimensions. The studies that I have initiated have instead been inspired by a neuroscientific model of working memory, in which I envisioned it as a complex of neurons, synapses, and brain areas. Innumerable studies showed how training modifies brain activity and nerve cells; why would there be something magical about the neurons that determine our working memory capacity?

Training probably only affects the areas that it activates. There is no training that magically improves the whole brain and all its functions. But if an area is responsible for many types of working memory tasks as well as the control of attention, which the mnemonic map in the parietal cortex seems to be, it might be worth spending time developing it. So along with Helena Westerberg, Hans Forssberg, Jonas Beckeman, and David Sjölander, I developed a computerized method of training working memory that is now being tested in scientific studies by us and independent groups around the world.

In several controlled studies we have seen how working memory training improves the performance of subjects by fifteen to twenty percent when they are tested on tasks extraneous to the

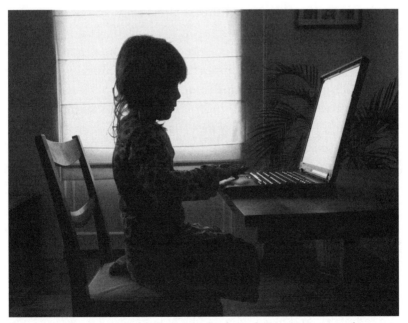

Computerized training of working memory has been shown to increase working memory capacity.

training program.[5,6] Moreover, the improvement is still there three and six months after the training period.[6] In one study I conducted with Lisa Thorell at Karolinska Institutet, we trained five-year-olds using only visuospatial exercises without numbers, letters, or words.[7] After the training period they were also better at exclusively lexical working memory tests, which indicates a capacity improvement that spreads across different kinds of stimuli.

In one study conducted by an independent group at Britain's York University under Joni Holmes and Susan Gathercole, it was found that training using our method improved performance on a battery of self-devised working memory tests, and that the effect persisted six months after training.[8] The study was interesting both in terms of how they selected their participants and of the tests they used to evaluate the effect. Instead of selecting children on the grounds of a particular diagnosis (e.g., attention-deficit/hyperactivity disorder [ADHD]), they simply measured the working memory of over 300 children and included the lowest performing fifteenth percentile. These children were then randomly assigned to receive either a real or "placebo" version of the training program.

One of the tests they used was the "classroom analog test." Now working memory is important for remembering instructions, such as "Go up to your room, put your socks on, and get your backpack," as well as all the instructions that we more or less explicitly give ourselves every day, such as "Start up your computer, send an email to your colleague, attach the article." Gathercole has devised a test for measuring precisely how good children are at remembering instructions using a variety of props (pencils, erasers, rulers, folders, boxes) in a range of colors (blue, yellow, red). The children are then given instructions as to what to do with them ("Place the red pencil in the yellow file"), which are gradually made longer and more complex ("Place the blue eraser and the red ruler in the blue box") until the children can no longer cope with them and give up ("Take the yellow and blue eraser and the red pencil and place them in the blue file, which you are then to place in the yellow box"). The test is designed to mimic the kind of tasks that schoolchildren are asked to perform daily, and here, too, the training group improved over the controls. This is an important discovery, not only because the instruction test is far removed from the tasks performed in the training program, which shows that the spreading effect is a genuine one, but also because it's a more realistic test of what we use working memory for in real life. Hopefully, the children derived a certain degree of benefit from it in their classroom, even if they do have only one color of eraser.

As we have already seen, working memory is closely associated with number sense and mathematical reasoning, in part via the parietal mnemonic map, and with this in mind Holmes and Gathercole also gave their subjects a test of mathematical reasoning. Immediately after training they observed no performance improvement in the children; six months later, however, they found statistically significant gains, suggesting the gradual enhancement of mathematical skills by a higher working memory capacity.[8]

It's never easy to measure the effects of training on daily behavior. However, for one study we gave out a list of questions about the defining behaviors of ADHD, such as difficulties in task completion and mind wandering, and found that the parents of children in the training group rated their children as much more attentive in their daily life than previously. The effects of working memory training on behavior have also been replicated by several studies conducted in the United States.[9,10]

One particularly interesting method of measuring behavior was used by Chloe Green and Julie Schweitzer at the University of California, Davis.[11] The children in the study, all of whom had an ADHD diagnosis, were placed in a test room designed like a classroom and asked to perform a task without letting themselves be disturbed by the other children or the objects around them. Their behavior was filmed by hidden cameras placed behind two-way mirrors. Every fifteen-second sequence of film was then assessed against a chart with respect to sitting still, concentrating on the task, daydreaming, fiddling, and so on by a panel blind to which children belonged to the group that had followed the real test program and that belonged to the "placebo" group. The teachers were also asked to assess the children's ADHD symptoms on a questionnaire.

On analyzing the results of the teachers' assessments, Green and Schweitzer noted no differences between the groups; on broadening their analysis to the panel's assessments, however, they found that the children in the training group performed significantly better than the control group in the aggregate measure of all types of "unfocused" behavior, the most salient gains being in "on task behavior" (i.e., subtle—but critical—behaviors, such as looking at the task in hand rather than out of the window). The effects of training are consistent with other studies showing that working memory capacity is linked to "remembering what to concentrate on" rather than daydreaming or letting the mind wander.[12]

Although most studies of working memory training have included children with ADHD, the effects appear to be general: if you're able to do focused training you'll also see improvements, no matter how old you are or what your concentration difficulties stem from.

As described in the story of Laura in Chapter 2, children who have undergone cancer therapies often develop serous cognitive problems and working memory impairments. Kristina Hardy, a pediatric neurologist from Duke University, has spent many years working with such children, and in an effort to find a method that could help them she contacted us to inquire about working memory training. Working with a group of children who had been treated for cancer and who all displayed problems similar to Laura's, she found that those who had been given working memory training not only showed performance gains on tests of working memory and attention compared to controls but also received higher ratings from their parents on assessments of daily-life management and cognitive abilities.

THE ART OF TRAINING

Exercises can be good—if you do them. How many of us are fully aware that a little physical exercise a few times a week is good for us but still fail to live up to our good intentions? It's not uncommon for people to fork out a king's ransom for a gym card, year after year, only to work out there a handful of times. "Next term I'll . . ." Motivation problems in following through training programs very much apply to cognitive training, too.

When we first saw the initial positive results of working memory training in controlled studies a few years ago, we wanted to test how training could work in practice. We got in touch with ten families who were keen to discover whether the training program could help their children, all of whom had some sort of concentration difficulty, and sent them a CD containing the program, which they were to use for twenty-five days' training over a period of five weeks. Since their results were logged automatically on their computers and sent via Internet to a server, we were able to monitor their progress. Not one single child completed the twenty-five-day program! The practical problems with cognitive training are not just a little practical problem but a gigantic practical problem.

With a little trial and error, we have gradually arrived at a method combining the right information with a reward scheme and a personal trainer that has encouraged children to complete the program as intended. At US clinics, where the method is used primarily for children with ADHD, over ninety percent of the young trainees now complete the entire program using this procedure.

The working memory training method that my colleagues and I have developed is currently used at roughly 200 clinics in the United States and Canada, and about twenty other countries.*

---

* The program is sold by a company called Cogmed, which is owned by Pearson Clinical Assessment. Since there are commercial interests involved, I should disclose that I remain employed at Karolinska Institutet, where I conduct research about cognitive training. I also work as a consultant for take out Cogmed/Pearson in the development of the training program, but I receive no royalties or other payment based on the sale or use of the program, and I have no options or shares in the company.

Around the world, teachers and psychologists have developed practical ways of implementing the training program. At a conference in Austin, Texas, I once listened to Rob Budwig talk about his experiences with working memory training in a school in Hydesville, California, where he works as a special needs teacher. Hydesville is a small upstate town with high unemployment, a relatively high proportion of mobile homes, and marijuana cultivation as one of the few growth businesses. The school in which he works has serious problems with truancy, weapons, and drugs. He was the only teacher there who used the method, and due to time constraints he had to train several students concurrently, so he built small booths separated by screens to prevent the children distracting each other.

Reward and feedback proved essential. Gold stars were pasted on a wall schedule to show how far each child had progressed in the program, this schedule being the first and last thing the pupils would check when they went to the training room every day. Rewards were small, practical things: post-it notes, string, or duct tape. However, the process was not without its complications. Rob recalls how one afternoon he was sitting at his desk when there came a loud knocking at his door. On opening, he was greeted by a student whose arms and legs were bound tight in the very duct tape he'd been given as a reward. He'd had to use his head to knock on the door.

Rob hasn't done any empirical study but from what he's seen in his students and what he's heard from their parents and other teachers, he's pleased with the results. But his expectations are starting from a very low level. One of the boys he trained had been reprimanded for hitting another child. But the teacher who reported the incident was pleased nonetheless, since after the training he could at least verbalize what had made him so angry. Rob continued to train his children in Hydesville, but the rewards no longer included duct tape.

My team has also carried out experiments to find out what happens in the brain when someone trains his or her working memory. In one study where we studied brain activity with a MR scanner before and after training, we found that training boosted activity in the parietal lobe and prefrontal cortext.[13] In Chapter 2 (see Fig. 2.3), we saw that these are the areas that are activated during different types of working memory task as well as during tasks that demand controlled attention. The parietal cortex is also where the mnemonic map resides, which could explain the improvements in math skills that Holmes and Gathercole recorded. Our functional magnetic resonance imaging studies also show how the areas that are associated with higher cognitive faculties are susceptible to training.

In a later study by Lars Nyberg's group at Umeå University, it was found that changes in the activity of the basal ganglia can be a key determinant in the training effect.[14] The basal ganglia are relay stations that unite large parts of the cortex and the thalamus, and are thus a critical brain structure. They are also important to our ability to sift out relevant information from surrounding noise, which is one aspect of both controlled attention and working memory.

In a subsequent study we used a positron emission tomography (PET) scanner to study whether training could also affect neuronal receptors.[15] The principle for PET is the bonding of a substance tagged with a radioactive isotope with a particular kind of receptor. The scanner then produces an image of where the radioactive substance accumulates, giving an indication of the number of receptors there are in that particular area. We were interested in dopamine receptors, which have long been known to be involved in working memory. The dopamine receptor is also interesting because disruption to the dopamine system can be a contributory factor to the problems associated with ADHD. The results of our study showed that the degree of improvement after working memory training correlated with changes to the density of cortical dopamine D1 receptors. This PET study was interesting because it shows that training not only affects the activity of neurons but also influences their fundamental biochemistry—something that had not previously been observed. It also demonstrates that the relationship between brain biochemistry and function is a mutual one: the brain's biochemistry affects behavior, but behavior can also affect the biochemistry.

A number of studies have been published recently that have used different kinds of working memory training. For instance, Lars Nyberg, Lars Bäckman, and collaborators have used a special kind of working memory test designed to assess the ability to update information in working memory, in which subjects are presented with a sequence of colors, numbers, or letters and then asked to recall the last four items shown. Training seems to have a certain effect on these tasks, but one that pertains mainly to other "updating" working memory tasks. There are as yet no studies regarding the effects it has on everyday attention or studies on children.[16]

Another study by Susanne Jaeggi, John Jonides, and collaborators examined the effect of training two working memory tasks simultaneously.[17] For this experiment, the researchers relayed a spoken number to the participants while showing them a circle on a computer screen in front of them. On the presentation of successive numbers and circles, the participants were asked to state whether the number or position of each circle was the same as the preceding number or position, a task that was made progressively harder as the length of the sequence to be memorized increased. After several weeks' training, it was found that the participants were able to perform better on a problem-solving task, but the extent to which the result was due to expectation effects is hard to judge as the study, unfortunately, used only a passive control group. But what was interesting about it was that the researchers used different groups and different periods of training, and that improvements in the subjects' reasoning ability were largely proportional to the amount of training they had received, although it took roughly eight hours of training for any significant results to manifest themselves.

CAN EVERYTHING BE TRAINED?

Studies of working memory training show that cognitive functions can improve through training. The principle that all functions can benefit from training ought to be a general one, but there can still be practical matters that make some functions more responsive to training than others, and that the transfer to improvement on other tasks differs depending on the type of training used. A reminder of this was an interesting study in which we tried—in vain, it has to be said—to train inhibitory ability.

Inhibitory ability is the ability to resist an impulse, a habit, or a movement that has already begun. If, for example, you're sitting in your car at a red light, and the light in the lane beside you turns green, your automatic response could be to step on the accelerator. The inhibitory ability is what hopefully prevents you from carrying through this action. A lack of this ability is a problem for many individuals, and there are theories that it's one of the key contributors to ADHD. There are good reasons, therefore, to try to find a method that can strengthen the inhibitory ability.

For the study, which was led by Lisa Thorell and me, we took children between four and five years old without any particular cognitive problems.[7] We then divided them into four groups: a group that trained inhibition, a group that trained working memory, a group that played a computer game, and a passive control group. The children in the inhibition group gradually improved their performance, but when we measured whether the training program had had any impact on tasks that it had not included we found that there were no transfer to other tasks at all. The children who had undergone the same degree of working memory training, however, saw gains on several untrained tasks involving working memory and concentration ability. So it seems as if the inhibitory ability might thus be more resistant to training; perhaps this is because the inhibition of an impulse is such a brief activity, lasting just a few hundred milliseconds, that it can never receive sufficient training.

There is still some doubt as to whether working memory training improves reasoning skills, with some studies yielding positive results, others negative, depending on the group being trained and how powers of reasoning are measured. In one study, led by Sissela Bergman Nutley, we tried to train reasoning ability simply by presenting 100 four-year-olds, divided into groups, with a string of problems at a reasonable level of difficulty for their age group.[18] One group trained reasoning skills and, compared with a control group that had worked with an ineffective computer program, exhibited performance enhancements not only on the kind of problems they had been training but also on several other reasoning tasks. This was just the first study, but a promising one nonetheless.

Games could be an optimal way to train cognitive faculties. One method using games is based on the developmental theories of Russian neuropsychologist Lev Vygotsky. The hypothesis is that children learn to control their behavior by gradually internalizing instructions, often with the help of external aids. For instance, a child learns to handle problems by hearing an adult's instructions, until eventually the child's behavior is controlled wholly by his or her own mind. A training method, called *Tools of the Mind*, has been devised to train this type of control through play. One such exercise might be for the children to pair off, and while one child reads a story holding a picture of a mouth, the other is to listen while holding a picture of an ear, the idea being that these external tools will help the children control their behavior. A randomized study showed that the method is effective, at least when it comes to children's ability to control their behavior in a classroom situation; unfortunately, however, it didn't include an active control group.[19]

MUSIC

In the 1990s, researchers showed that if people listen to Mozart, they perform better on tests of spatial awareness. The phenomenon, which was dubbed the "Mozart effect," prompted volumes of follow-up studies and a plethora of commercial products, such as Baby Genius CDs with selected works of Mozart for ambitious parents to play to their infants. The Mozart effect proved hard to replicate. There's nothing magical about Mozart's notes; his music might have a certain benefit, but it has everything to do with the general effects of all mood-lifting, soothing music and nothing to do with the mathematical structure of his compositions. However, the Baby Genius CDs continue to sell.

Having said this, there is growing evidence that learning a musical instrument has a positive effect on cognitive ability. Several studies have shown that children who take music lessons also perform better at tests of spatial awareness, memory, reading, and math. The problem with many of the studies is that children who take music lessons tend to come from more educated families with more ambitious parents. So it's hard to say whether the musical lessons actually are the determining factor.

In an attempt to find this out, Glenn Schellenberg of the University of Toronto conducted a study in which he randomly assigned six-year-olds into two groups, one that received music lessons and one that received drama lessons.[20] The music lessons were held for groups of six children, who received professional instruction in either singing or playing the piano. When the researchers tested the children after a year with thirty-six weeks of teaching, they found that the children from the music group outperformed those from the drama group on tests of IQ. However, although the effects were broad rather than for a specific cognitive function, they were also rather weak and corresponded to roughly a three percentage point improvement on the IQ tests compared with controls.

Learning to play a musical instrument requires daily concentrated training, training in keeping brief passages in working memory and fixing longer passages in the long-term memory. If you lose concentration, you get immediate feedback in that you hear the wrong note. It's probably these demands that produced the side effects in all the tests in which gains were observed. The researchers thus didn't interpret the effect as being specific to music but as the result of the cognitive components of learning, and argued that a similar result would have been produced from any other concentration-demanding activity, such as playing chess.

Our Nynäshamn study didn't only involve giving children tests of cognitive ability to perform; we also gave their parents questionnaires about their children's hobbies, including whether they played a musical instrument. On reassessing their cognitive abilities two years later, Sissela Bergman Nutley, who led the analysis, found that the children who played an instrument had improved between the first and second tests more than their nonmusical peers, on both working memory and reasoning tasks; these results held even when we controlled for factors such as parental education, and thus they support the theory that making music can boost cognitive abilities.[21]

Computer games are not only the primary interest of increasing numbers of children but also the target of much serious scientific attention. One much-discussed study, which was published in *Nature* in 2003, showed that people who spend a lot of time playing computer games perform better on tests requiring rapid perceptual responses. Ten hours' training playing an action game (like Medal of Honor) led to a greater performance improvement in perceptual processing than did a similar period of training playing a control game (Tetris).[22] The results, however, later proved to be unreliable. When another team from the University of Illinois tried to replicate the study using the same games but twice as many participants and double the training period, they could see no significant effects of the action game.[23]

In our study of the Nynäshamn children, we were also interested in studying the effects of computer games. We tested working memory, mathematical skills, and reading skills with a two-year interval, and on both occasions asked parents to rate how much time their children spent at their games consoles, and the parents and teachers to rate their degree of concentration difficulties. A Master's dissertation by Douglas Sjövall showed that computer games induced no impairments in the children who played computer games or any observable deterioration in concentration abilities; on the contrary, there was in fact a weak but nonetheless positive tendency toward an improvement in both parameters measured.

What became of the subjects in the BBC's "Brain Training" study? When the thousands of participants were tested after six weeks of training, no significant difference was observed between the groups.[1] How can we then reconcile these results with those showing the effects of cognitive training, including that of working memory?

One explanation is that concepts such as "brain training" are far too broad and nebulous. After all, no one would dream of conducting a study to find out whether "medicine" generally works or whether "food" is healthy. If a pharmaceutical study shows a certain drug to be ineffective, no one draws the conclusion that medicines are useless against disease. There are a great many factors that must be specified when we talk of cognitive training, such as exactly which functions are being trained, how the degree of difficulty is pitched to the subject group, how much time the participants spend training every day, the total length of the training period, the quality of the training, and how its effects are measured.

For the BBC study, the participants were asked to train for ten minutes a day, three days a week, making a total training period of four hours. The studies that had previously demonstrated the effectiveness of training used at least eight hours. In our studies of working memory training, the children carry out twelve to fifteen hours of training. The training time alone can in this case explain the lack of effect. However, there are other problems with the British study, such as the fact that the participants' training was unmonitored and that we know nothing of the quality of the programs. But negative findings can also give us interesting information: for example, it takes intensive, prolonged training with some kind of quality control for any effect to be had. Routine training for ten minutes a day a few days a week produces no results. This is not actually that surprising. No one would expect to develop an athlete's cardiovascular fitness by walking ten minutes a day three times a week. Some forms of training are more effective, others less so. But many training exercises can deliver—if you do them, that is.

CHAPTER 10

༄

Body and Soul

Every day, the children at Naperville Central High School near Chicago put on their heart rate monitors before the day's physical education lesson. On occasion, it involves a two-kilometer run. However, it's not how quickly they complete the course that's important; it's the effort they put into running it, as revealed by the monitor. The heart rate can be expressed in terms of a percentage of the maximum pulse, whereby eighty percent or more of maximum is ideal for increasing oxygen uptake. The pupils naturally differ in terms of muscle strength and oxygen uptake capacity, but in expressing performance as a percentage of maximum heart rate, the teacher can confirm that everyone has at least tried. Each child competes against his or her own results, and as long as the child improves he or she gets higher grades.

This school has been a pioneer in designing physical exercise programs for school children. The programs were the brainchild of a physical education teacher in response to the alarming statistics showing that children are becoming progressively overweight. Thirty percent of all children in the United States are judged to be overweight, six times more than in 1980. The corresponding figure in many European countries is lower, but still some twenty percent of teenagers fall into the overweight bracket.

What makes the Naperville program noteworthy is not only that it has increased the amount of training but also that it focuses on cardiovascular training rather than specific sports. And it's the heart rate monitors that have proved to be the key to its success. Today, only one percent of the children in Naperville Central High are overweight—which is a partial victory—but above all it's the effect the program is having on classroom performance that has caught the attention of researchers. The Naperville pupils are top performers on national tests not only in the United States but also in international comparisons. Other schools inspired by Naperville have also seen positive results. A school in Titusville, Pennsylvania, introduced a similar reform to its physical education program and invested in workout machines, climbing walls, exercise bikes, and heart rate monitors. They dropped the amount of traditional teaching in favor of physical exercise, and since the trial started the children's performances have shot up from below the state average, to sixteen percent above in reading tests and seventeen percent above in math. In another school in Kansas City with children from low socioeconomic status areas (as illustrated by the fact that they are entitled to free school lunches), the amount of physical exercise was raised from one session a week to forty-five minutes a day. The most salient effect that has subsequently been measured is a huge year-on-year drop in "discipline incidents" from 228 to 95.

The results from Naperville and the other schools are not from controlled studies. Naperville is an extremely affluent suburb and the children there would have performed well even without any extra training initiatives. This said, an ever-growing body of research is demonstrating how physical exercise is good not only for raising the cardiovascular fitness and lowering the weight but also for improving cognitive skills (see Fig. 10.1). And now we're starting to glimpse the brain mechanisms that are responsible for these improvements.

JOGGING AND THE BRAIN

It has long been known that older people in a relatively good state of health also perform better on a range of psychological tests, especially ones relating to reaction time, than their more

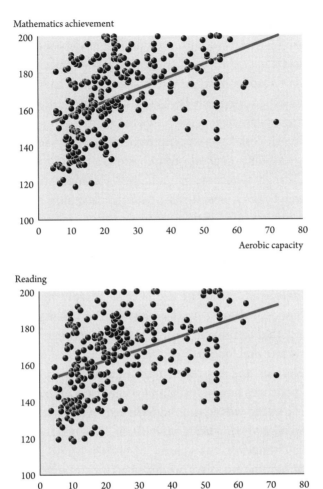

Figure 10.1 The fitness levels of schoolchildren (measured as aerobic capacity) versus performance on tests of mathematical and reading skills (from Hillman et al., 2008).[4]

sedentary peers. This has previously been interpreted as a general effect of a more efficient oxygen uptake bringing more oxygen-rich blood to the brain. An increasing number of studies are now demonstrating that the benefits of physical fitness relate not only to the elderly and reaction time but much more so to memory and reasoning skills; and that they're not simply the result of greater oxygen metabolism but of a direct modification of the brain's nerve cells.

Arthur Kramer from Illinois University is one of the leading researchers in this field, and as a former professional boxer he possibly has a vested interest in studying the effects of training. In a series of studies, Kramer and his colleagues have shown how the effects of training can be measured using a magnetic resonance scanner. His first study involved participants who underwent a fitness test before being randomly assigned to either a training group or a control group.[1] The training group were put through a range of aerobic fitness exercises, most notably power walks, three times a week for six months, and sure enough their level of cardiovascular fitness improved by roughly ten percent. The control group did stretching exercises for the same period of time, which, as expected, had little impact on their overall state of fitness. The researchers measured the brain activity of all participants before and after the six months of training as they performed a concentration-demanding task. Comparing the results, they found that aerobic training boosted activity in both the frontal and parietal lobes.

Later, Kramer and his team used a similar training program consisting of three hours' training a week for six months.[2] Again, the training group was compared with a stretching control group, but instead of analyzing brain activity, they turned their attention to possible changes in the volume of gray or white matter. They found that aerobic training produced a thickening of the cortex in several places, including the frontal lobe. Six months was thus enough to produce an observable degree of cortical growth.

Ana Pereira of Columbia University in New York studied the effects of training on people between the ages of twenty-one and forty-five.[3] Pereira's team put the participants on a three-month training program, and during each of the four-times-weekly sessions pushed them close to the limit of their peak oxygen uptake. They also gave them long-term memory tasks to perform and measured the blood volume in different parts of their hippocampus before and after each session. There was no control group in the study, but improvements in the oxygen uptake capacity of the participants varied, correlating with improvements in working memory and increases in blood volume to the hippocampus.

In the second part of the study, the researchers put mice through a similar training program and compared them with a passive control group. Here, too, they found an increase in blood volume to the hippocampus that correlated with the formation of new neurons.

There are numerous studies on the effect of physical exercise on the animal brain. Some of the most robust findings are that training increases cell formation in the hippocampus and stimulates the secretion of growth factors named with a thicket of abbreviations such as IGF-1, VEGF, FGF, HGF, and BDNF.[4] Here we see some familiar faces. The gyrus dentatus is the part of the hippocampus where cell formation takes place. More prolific cell formation is associated with better long-term memory encoding and is seen in children as well as in rats living in cages full of toys and rats raised by caring mothers. And the effects of enriched environments and caring mothers could be measured in terms of brain-derived neurotrophic factor (BDNF) production. Thus, the mechanisms for what is good for the memory and the individual coincide very closely, regardless of their causes. In many cases, the positive effects resemble the circumstances that pertain more to those of the child or young adult. The amount of BDNF, for example, decreases with age, and in one study it was shown that the decline in BDNF in individuals over sixty explained their poorer performance on a working memory test, even after having controlled for the fact that BDNF and working memory both deteriorate with age.[5] Fitness training is thus one method for keeping the brain young.

We don't yet know exactly how hard the training should be or how often one has to train for observable cognitive improvements to be attained. Physiologically, experts usually maintain that it's chiefly intensive training that improves oxygen uptake and that we should therefore train at eighty percent, at least, of our maximum heart rate. The maximum heart rate varies from individual to individual, but a rule of thumb is that you can obtain your HRmax (as it's known) by subtracting your age from 220. A twenty-year old thus has an HRmax of roughly 200, and should train with a heart rate above 160.

In his book *Spark*, Dr. John Ratey from Harvard Medical School sums up the effects of physical exercise, which, among other benefits, improves classroom performance and reduces stress and depression.[6] His condensed training recipe is to do intensive training four times a week, to a degree specified in terms of calories per kilo body weight. When I applied the formula to myself, I calculated that if I was to follow his recommendations, I'd have to run five kilometers, four times a week, with a mean heart rate of over 150 beats per minute. I must admit there aren't that many weeks of the year when I achieve this dose of exercise. But after reading his book and the research on the cognitive benefits of training, I've definitely been inspired to put my jogging shoes on more often.

If you baulk at such a training regime, I should add that not all researchers are of the same opinion. It's an open question whether the same principles—that eighty percent of the HRmax raises oxygen uptake—also applies to an escalation of BDNF. Several studies seem to suggest that the effect happens gradually; while it's true that the more often and more intensively you train, the better the results, even at a low level of intensity training is still worthwhile. In one study, the effects of thirty-minute training sessions using two different degrees of intensive training were compared in young adults. The high intensive group trained at around eighty-five percent of their HRmax (corresponding to 150 beats per minute), the low intensive group at seventy percent (122 beats per minute). The researchers duly recorded a thirty percent increase of BDNF in the high intensive group but also a ten percent increase in the low intensive group.[7]

We cannot say for certain whether the effects of exercise in children are the same as those found in adults. However, in a review of studies on the effects on children between the ages of four to eighteen, a positive effect was found on almost all parameters measured: perception, verbal skills, reasoning skills, and math.[8] The effects seemed to be very broad, in other words, and not confined to one particular function. Moreover, the statistics suggest that physical fitness also benefits classroom performance. Data collected by the California Department of Education on the fitness levels of school children in the state and their exam results exhibit a clear correlation between fitness and performance in both math and reading, but not between muscle strength or agility and classroom performance, indicating once again that it's fitness training that's the key to improving memory and cognition (see Fig. 10.1).[4]

I should mention here that there are still very few controlled studies of the effects of training in children. Reviews of research in the field suggest that its impact on cognition is weaker than it is in adults (including the elderly), possibly by as much as fifty percent.[4] On a comparison of individuals, like that from the California Department of Education, it also seems as if the strongest relationship exists in the lowest performing children. This could mean that sedentary children have much to gain from training up to an average level of fitness, but beyond that the gains aren't that significant.

However, despite all the question marks, all available results point in the same direction: aerobic fitness training has a positive effect on cognitive ability and classroom performance. The advantage of physical exercise is that its effects seem to be so broad, and in addition to enhancing a number of cognitive functions it also reduces excess weight and stress. Most schools should ultimately increase the amount of fitness training they give their pupils and students, even if it is at the expense of other subjects.

Plato wrote: "In order for man to succeed in life, God provided him with two means, education and physical activity. Not separately, one for the soul and the other for the body, but for the two together. With these two means, man can attain perfection."

The association between physical and cognitive functions is thus by no means new, even if Plato did have little to say about BDNF.

INTELLIGENCE AND INFECTIONS

Knowledge of how physical training and stress affect children's cognitive abilities illustrates just how many factors contribute to human development. An individual's mental and physical health often go hand in hand with cognitive function. It will be interesting to see what effect physical training will have in combination with cognitive training. One hypothesis is that the former will stimulate neuron production by boosting BDNF, allowing the latter to make use of and optimize the function of the new nerve cells thus produced. In the enriched environment studies, we have also seen that the effect of physical training can be augmented by a more stimulating environment.

Diet and sleep are other factors that play a part in the context. A better diet not only leads to a more even blood sugar level but also aids physical training. Physical training reduces stress levels and improves sleep, which in turn is crucial to the function of working memory, long-term memory, and attention. I once heard a teacher say, "Just give me children who've had nine hours' sleep and a proper breakfast every day, and I'll show you that we can raise the mean score on standard assessment tests by twenty percent."

When it comes to diet, many parents seem keen to ply their children with beneficial oils, mainly omega-3 fatty acids. Omega-3 fatty acids are an essential component of myelin, the fat that sheathes the axons in the white matter. So the idea that a lack of fatty acids could influence brain function is not that crazy; however, the results of studies on the effects of omega oils are not yet unequivocal. In one oft-cited study, children with pronounced motor problems and clumsiness and a diagnosis of developmental coordination disorder were randomly divided into a treatment group that received six capsules containing a mix of omega-3 and omega-6 oils, and a control group that received the same amount of olive oil.[9] After three months, the researchers saw no effect on their motor symptoms, although the treatment group did perform better on tests of reading ability and spelling. However, several studies of children with attention-deifcit/hyperactivity disorder have observed no change in symptoms or improvements in memory and attention after taking omega-3 fatty acids.[10,11] It's possible that such fatty acids can have an effect on certain subgroups of children, or on children of a certain age, or that you need the right dose and blend of oils. But one thing's for sure: stuffing six fish oil capsules down your children every day doesn't seem to be the most direct route to the top of the class.

Globally speaking, it's not the question of the optimal dose of omega-3 that's keeping parents awake at night. For many families in the third world, it's about having access to food, clean water, and health care. And this is not only a matter of their survival. A study from 2010 led by Christopher Eppig at the University of New Mexico indicates that infections can be the most critical factor affecting the maturation of the brain.[12]

The researchers studied national variations in the results of intelligence tests, on which many African countries score particularly poorly. The cause of these differences is an old and controversial question, and it has been attributed to everything from genes and temperature to level of education and differences in how cultures prepare people for taking specifically American-designed IQ tests. In an effort to examine whether the incidence of disease, infections particularly, was a possible explanation, Eppig accessed World Health Organization statistics on the number of disease years caused by the twenty-eight most common infections. Data are available for 192 counties, and for many African countries the list is topped by diarrhea, caused often by the lack of clean drinking water.

On comparing these disease statistics with average performance on intelligence tests, for which data were available for 142 countries, he found that the two measures were highly correlated, the degree of infection explaining sixty-eight percent of the differences in mean test scores between the countries. The correlation was present when all countries were included and when the comparison was confined to countries in Africa, Asia, and the Pacific region. The correlation with infections was the strongest of all variables tested, and it could not be dismissed as an effect of educational level, malnourishment, or gross domestic product.

The study is a controversial one, but it is not inconceivable that infections would influence the maturation of the brain. Brain development, as we saw in Chapter 2, is extremely energy demanding. The brain of a neonate, in which new synapses are created every second, devours no less than eighty-five percent of the baby's energy; in a five-year-old, it consumes forty-four percent and in a ten-year-old it still accounts for roughly thirty-three percent of the body's total energy needs. An infection can be a great drain on the body's energy for several reasons, one because the immune defence is highly energy-demanding, another because those that cause diarrhea also cause malnourishment. Parasites can also directly consume the body's organs. If the body, when thus infected, redistributes its energy to fuel its immune defence, it's likely that brain development will be compromised.

Education is a narrow term that merely conjures up images of classrooms. What we're really interested in, however, is child development, and this includes both body *and* mind, knowledge *and* health. *Mens sana in corpore sano*—a sound mind in a sound body.

CHAPTER 11

❧

This Will Change Everything

If you do a search for scientific articles on "learning" and "brain," you'll find over 80,000 such papers published since 1945. Of these, eighty percent will have been published after 1990 and fifty percent since 2000. We are in the midst of a swelling torrent of knowledge about learning.

One of the 5,000 articles on learning and the brain that came out in 2009 was titled "Foundations for a New Science of Learning"[1] and was published in *Science*, one of the most prestigious of scientific periodicals. In it, the authors argue that we're seeing a merging of knowledge from neuroscience, psychology, pedagogy, and information technology that's set to give rise to a new era of learning. For a number of years, experimental psychology and brain science have been unified into a research field known as cognitive neuroscience; pedagogy, on the other hand, still lives very much its own life. It is time to unite, for educational scientists to take on board the discoveries of cognitive neuroscience and for pedagogical issues and experience to direct the experimental work done by cognitive neuroscientists.

One interesting idea for how to bring researchers together and make them focus their efforts is to announce a prize. In 1996, the X-Prize organization announced an award of ten million dollars for the person who could construct an aeroplane able to carry people to the outer edges of the Earth's atmosphere (and bring them back alive), twice in two weeks. In 2006, a team of researchers claimed the prize and flew a plane to almost weightless altitudes a hundred kilometers up. The challenge not only resulted in a new type of aircraft but also kicked off a small private aerospace industry, a commercial field that had never before existed.

The success of the initiative has led to a string of similar prizes. The company Netflix, which distributes films via the Internet, is offering a million dollars to the person who can find a better algorithm than theirs for suggesting new films based on a customer's previous ratings; the US defense organization DARPA has announced a prize to whomever can construct a driverless car that can negotiate city traffic; Virgin has promised twenty-five million dollars to the inventor of a method for absorbing greenhouse gases from the atmosphere.

Why not an X Prize for learning? A million dollars to the one who can find a better algorithm than what we currently have for how learning is to be optimally spaced out in time; ten million to those who can create a significantly better method for helping children with dyscalculia; and a hundred million to those who can create a scientifically based, digitalized form of elementary teaching that can be sent wirelessly to developing countries. The fact is that learning is one of the areas that the X-Prize organization is considering for the future, and it is welcoming submissions of proposals for a suitable challenge.

FIVE THEMES

As we await future progress and prizes, we can note that research has already made at least some headway, as I've tried to overview in this book. It's possible to pick out five themes, or fields, where cognitive neuroscience is influencing our view of child development and learning.

The first is the *map*. The human psyche has long been something of a black box, or, if you will, a car with its hood closed. Brain research allows us to open the hood and examine the engine. In its simplest version, the blueprint we get is kind of a map of the various functions residing in the brain. The map of mathematics areas enables us to understand why a prematurely born child can have problems subtracting but not learning the times tables by heart; our understanding of the role of the hippocampus explains why Jon (Chapter 4), while equipped with a serviceable working memory, cannot encode new long-term memories; and we can understand why problems such as dyslexia and dyscalculia are closely related.

However, the map does more than just explain; it can also be used as a means of *prediction* regarding which children might fall into the risk zone for various problems. This is the second theme, and it is a field in which cognitive neuroscience can make a solid contribution. If these children are to be helped, they must be identified in time before they lose years of schooling owing to an undiagnosed functional disability. And here we can already find methods that enable us to ascertain at an early stage whether a child risks developing reading and writing difficulties.

The third theme is *intervention*. Identifying children in the risk zone is only meaningful if there is some way of helping them. Methods are available for many such cognitive problems, particularly ones involving training. Knowledge of how the brain encodes numbers in a spatial dimension in the parietal lobe has spawned numerous methods for learning mathematics; and knowledge of an overlap between areas of attention and the varieties of working memory has led to a method of training working memory. Unfortunately, however, the application of neuroscientific knowledge to methodological development is still a relatively barren field, the lack of breakthroughs being attributable, in part, to the genuine ignorance that neuroscientists possess of pedagogy as a science and the points of inquiry it raises. Bridges need to be built.

The fourth theme is *sculpting*, which affects our views of human development. The brains of children and adolescents are not mini versions of the adult brain any more than sperm contain microscopic fetuses. The brain is shaped through decades of growing and pruning. How different parts of the brain mature explains the gradual development of faculties such as working memory, and the fact that we are born with a hippocampus that matures slowly by degrees possibly explains why you probably don't remember the color of the cot you slept in as a baby. The knowledge of sculpting can also show, as in the case of Laura (Chapter 2), what disruption of the normal development trajectory can entail—in much the same way as studies of the risk taking and emotional teenage brain show that it doesn't exist on a point halfway between childhood and adulthood, but at a stage subject to its own unique conditions.

The fifth theme is *plasticity*. The brain creates function, but our environment and our actions influence the brain. We've seen how the brain is shaped by working memory training and playing a musical instrument, and how levels of BDNF can be boosted by a few jogs around the park every week. Dopamine affects working memory, but working memory training can also influence the number of dopamine receptors. The hippocampus determines how the long-term memory develops, but a stimulating environment and opportunities for exploration and learning also affect the hippocampus. The simple fact that brain research has shown how plastic the brain is, is in itself extremely important. It gives inspiration and hope that cognitive difficulties can be compensated for.

A pattern that has gradually emerged in the process of writing this book is how the link between brain, function, and environment often gets caught in a circle, be it virtuous or vicious. Negative expectations, such as girls being worse at math than boys, creates a stress that does indeed cause girls to perform worse when placed in a group of boys and told that they are to have their mathematical skills evaluated. This inferior performance then reinforces the prejudices that exist about girls and math.

Similarly, poor classroom performance is one of the key stress factors for schoolchildren of all ages, and stress is one of the most negative determiners of classroom performance. The protracted stress that accompanies poverty impairs working memory, which in turn leads to worse classroom performance; and a lower level of education increases the risk of poverty for the next generation. Another example is how negligent mothers raise children who are stress-sensitive and who have poor long-term memories, and who in turn become negligent mothers themselves over their own stress-sensitive offspring.

The vicious-circle mechanisms can only be understood through knowledge of the functional map, sculpting, and plasticity. We can't understand how prejudices can become self-fulfilling prophecies if we don't understand how stress reactions affect nerve cells, how the effect on the nerve cells influences working memory, and how working memory is linked to mathematics and school performance. The protracted stress caused by poverty has a permanent impact on the brain through its equally protracted sculpting and it's because of the energy-demanding sculpting of the brain that infections are so detrimental to its development. But there is some light in all this gloom: if we know these mechanisms, we have a better chance of breaking the cycles.

Future learning will probably be shaped by a conglomeration of scientific disciplines: experimental psychology, cognitive neuroscience, pedagogy, and information technology. I am convinced that if we are to make any progress, it will only be through scientific method and randomized studies. Teaching has been dominated far too much by political opinion and trendy pedagogical whims. No teaching method suits all students, and adapting education to individual needs means not only being quick to catch and help children with difficulties but also providing those who are fully capable and who need extra stimulation with the resources and tools they need to develop to their full potential.

A SCHOOLGIRL OF THE FUTURE

Two hundred years ago, Jean-Jacques Rousseau described in his book *Émile* his version of the best conceivable education: personal instruction from a mentor who would contribute step by step to a child's development. *Émile* was a pure thought experiment. Rousseau himself wasn't a teacher, had no pupil, and didn't raise his own children. But since the book was published his ideas have been a source as much of inspiration as of criticism. Neal

Stephenson's *The Diamond Age—A Young Lady's Illustrated Primer* is arguably an *Émile* for the twenty-first century.[2]

Stephenson's novel is set at some time in the mid-twenty-first century. The protagonist, Nell, is a four-year-old girl from the slums, who chances across the most advanced teaching tool in existence: an interactive computer program, a kind of animated primer. The primer begins by telling Nell stories, which gradually introduce new concepts and become progressively complex as the girl's abilities and knowledge expand. Eventually the stories take on the character of adventure games in which she is given missions, and the learning comes more as a side effect of their completion. At the age of sixteen, Nell reaches the end of the book's adventures, and in one of her last missions she has to outwit a cruel king and learn the art of creating nanotechnological inventions. She builds her own "illustrated primer" and creates her own world of stories.

Stephenson's digital primer is a blend of personal mentor, Wikipedia, problem-based learning, and adventure game. In his previous books he has fantasized about phenomena that have since become reality—so who knows, maybe it won't be long before we see illustrated primers on the shelves of all good bookstores.

The final objective in Stephenson's tale is for Nell to create her own computer program, her own book, and her own worlds. This educational goal—to provide children with the tools they need to create themselves—reminds me of how developmental psychologist Jean Piaget looked upon the objective of child development. "Education, for most people, means trying to lead the child to resemble the typical adult . . . But for me, education means making creators . . . You have to make inventors, innovators, not conformists."[3]

Piaget was wrong about children and mathematics, but in this case I cannot but agree with him.

Chris Anderson is neither a scientist nor a teacher but an inspirational visionary. He is editor-in-chief of the magazine *Wired*, which was ahead of its time in describing how developments in information technology would shape our society, economy, and culture. Chris has written two books, is a popular speaker, and runs *TED*, a forum that invites speakers from all over the world to hold lectures that are then spread free on the Internet.

Chris Anderson outlined his vision of the future in *This Will Change Everything*, a book containing a collection of essays by authors, artists, scientists, and other intellectuals, each with their own idea about which invention or idea could radically change the world and human lives.[4] The book is packed with descriptions of new forms of solar energy, cures for cancer, life-prolonging medicines, and teleports that could transport our bodies from one place to another at lightning speed. In his essay, Chris maintains that's it's the education of the future that will really change the world.

The focus of his essay is on the role of information technology, which is natural given his background. But the computer is just a tool; it will not revolutionize education in and of itself—no more than the flannelboard or video did—and cannot unless we fill it with the right content. And this content will come from research into learning processes. I'm therefore taking Anderson's example to illustrate the importance of learning for the individual, too, and the intrinsic power that new forms of learning possess.

His essay invites us to carry out the following thought experiment: imagine a person who you think has made a profound impact on the world. It might be a composer whose music has spread joy, a poet or author who has inspired generations, a scientist who has discovered a cure, or an inventor whose new technologies have changed the way we live. Imagine, then, that this person had been born in a rural French village in the 1100s or in Ethiopia in the 1980s, with no education, no intellectual stimulation, and no ability to develop his mind and abilities. What contribution would he then have made to the world? Probably none at all. Imagine the world without this person's contribution. The difference between the two worlds is the value of his once having access to the right kind of stimulation and education. Millions of children today don't have such opportunities, and there in the undeveloped masses resides the latent potential that could change everything.

A girl born today, somewhere in southern Africa perhaps, might by the age of ten have the use of a laptop with a high-resolution touchscreen and wireless Internet for a fraction of the current cost. This little portable computer would then give her access to the best interactive teaching tools, the best scientifically developed learning methods, and the best lectures held by the best teachers. Maybe she will be the one to save the world for our grandchildren.

NOTES

CHAPTER 1

1. Nilsson, B. B. (2007). *Nej, jag är inte dum ... jag har bara lite otur när jag tänker.* Burgsvik, Sweden: Valar Press.
2. Kane, M. J., et al. (2007). For whom the mind wanders, and when: An experience-sampling study of working memory and executive control in daily life. *Psychological Science, 18,* 614–621.
3. Gathercole, S. E., & Alloway, T. P. (2008). Working memory and learning: A practical guide for teachers. Thousand Oaks, CA: Sage.
4. Alloway, T. P., et al. (2009). The cognitive and behavioral characteristics of children with low working memory. *Child Development, 80,* 606–621.
5. Kelly, K., & Ramundo, P. (2006). You mean I'm not lazy, stupid or crazy?! A self-help book for adults with attention deficit disorder. New York: Simon & Schuster.
6. Teach ADHD. (2010). Retrieved April 2012, from http://research. aboutkidshealth.ca/teachadhd/about

CHAPTER 2

1. Lagercrantz, H. (2005). *I barnets hjärna.* Stockholm: Bonnier Fakta.
2. Chugani, H. T., et al. (1987). Positron emission tomography study of human brain functional development. *Annals of Neurology, 22,* 487–497.
3. Shaw, P., et al. (2008). Neurodevelopmental trajectories of the human cerebral cortex. *Journal of Neuroscience, 28,* 3586–3594.
4. Giedd, J. N., et al. (1999). Brain development during childhood and adolescence: A longitudinal MRI study. *Nature Neuroscience, 2,* 861–863.
5. Shaw, P., et al. (2007). Attention-deficit/hyperactivity disorder is charcterized by a delay in cortical maturation. *Proceedings of the National Academy of Sciences USA, 104*(49), 19649–19654.
6. Castellanos, F. X., et al. (2002). Developmental trajectories of brain volume abnormalities in children and adolescents with attention-deficit/ hyperactivity disorder. *Journal of the American Medical Association, 288,* 1740–1748.

7. Friedman, N. P., et al. (2008). Individual differences in executive functions are almost entirely genetic in origin. *Journal of Experimental Psychology: General, 137,* 201–225.

8. Luciano, M., et al. (2001). Genetic covariance among measures of information processing speed, working memory, and IQ. *Behavioral Genetics, 31,* 581–592.

9. Dumontheil, I., et al. (2011). The influence of COMT genotype on working memory changes during adolescence. *Biological Psychiatry, 70*(3), 222–229.

10. Hubacek, J. A., et al. (2001). A possible role of apolipoprotein E polymorphism in predisposition to higher education. *Neuropsychobiology, 43,* 200–203.

11. Alexander, D. M., et al. (2007). The contribution of apolipoprotein E alleles on cognitive performance and dynamic neural activity over six decades. *Biological Psychology, 75,* 229–238.

12. Söderqvist, S., et al. (2010). The SNAP25 gene is linked to working memory capacity and maturation of the posterior cingulate cortex during childhood. *Biological Psychiatry, 68,* 1120–1125.

13. Nagy, Z., et al. (2004). Regional maturation of white matter during childhood and development of function. *Journal of Cognitive Neuroscience, 16,* 1227–1233.

14. Klingberg, T. (2006). Development of a superior frontal-intraparietal network for visuospatial working memory. *Neuropsychologia, 44,* 2171–2177.

15. Karlsgodt, K. H., et al. (2011). A multimodal assessment of the genetic control over working memory. *Journal of Neuroscience, 30*(24), 8197–8202.

16. Klingberg, T., et al. (2000). Microstructure of temporoparietal white matter as a basis for reading ability: Evidence from diffusion tensor magnetic resonance imaging. *Neuron, 25,* 493–500.

17. Maddrey, A. M., et al. (2005). Neuropsychological performance and quality of life of 10 year survivors of childhood medulloblastoma. *Journal of Neurooncology, 72,* 245–253.

CHAPTER 3

1. Somerville, L. H., & Casey, B. J. (2010). Developmental neurobiology of cognitive control and motivational systems. *Current Opinion in Neurobiology, 20,* 236–241.

2. van Leijonhorst, L., et al. (2010). What motivates the adolescent? Brain regions mediating reward sensitivity across adolescence. *Cerebral Cortex, 20,* 61–69.

3. Cohen, J. R., et al. (2010). A unique adolescent response to reward prediction errors. *Nature Neuroscience, 13,* 669–671.

4. Cauffman, E., et al. (2010). Age differences in affective decision making as indexed by performance on the Iowa Gambling Task. *Developmental Psychology, 46,* 193–207.

5. Yurgelun-Todd, D. A., & Killgore, W. D. (2006). Fear-related activity in the prefrontal cortex increases with age during adolescence: A preliminary fMRI study. *Neuroscience Letters, 406,* 194–199.
6. Bainbridge, D. (2009). *Teenagers—a natural history.* Toronto, ON: Greystone Books.

CHAPTER 4

1. Brown, A. L., & Scott, M. S. (1971). Recognition memory for pictures in preschool children. *Journal of Experimental Child Psychology, 11,* 401–412.
2. Baker-Ward, L., & Ornstein, P. A. (1988). Age differences in visual-spatial memory performance: Do children really outperform adults when playing concentrations? *Bulletin of the Psychonomic Society, 26,* 331–332.
3. Gulya, M., et al. (2002). The development of explicit memory for basic perceptual features. *Journal of Experimental Child Psychology, 81,* 276–297.
4. Goswami, U. (2008). *Cognitive development—the learning brain.* East Sussex, UK: Psychology Press.
5. Obituary. (2008, December 20). *The Economist,* p. 134.
6. Richmond, J., & Nelson, C. A. (2007). Accounting for change in declarative memory: A cognitive neuroscience perspective. *Developmental Review, 27,* 349–373.
7. Gould, E., et al. (1999). Hippocampal neurogenesis in adult Old World primates. *Proceedings of the National Academy of Sciences USA, 96,* 5263–5267.
8. Tang, Y. P., et al. (1999). Genetic enhancement of learning and memory in mice. *Nature, 401,* 63–69.
9. Landauer, T. K., & Bjork, R. A. (1978). Optimum rehearsal patterns and name learning. In M. M. Gruneberg, P. E. Morris, & R. N. Sykes (Eds.), *Practical aspects of memory.* San Diego, CA: Academic Press.
10. Wolf, G. (2008, April 21). Want to remember everything you'll ever learn? Surrender to this algorithm, *Wired.* Retrieved April 2012, from http://www.wired.com/medtech/health/magazine/16-05/ff_wozniak?currentPage=all
11. Brandt, K. R., et al. (2008). Impairment of recollection but not familiarity in a case of developmental amnesia. *Neurocase, 15,* 60–65.
12. BBC. (2008). How does your memory work? [television program]. London: BBC.

CHAPTER 5

1. Tammet, D. (2008). *Born on a blue day.* New York: Free Press.
2. Dehaene, S., et al. (1993). The mental representation of parity and numerical magnitude. *Journal of Experimental Psychology: General, 122,* 371–396.

3. Dehaene, S., et al. (1990). Is numerical comparison digital? Analogical and symbolic effects in two-digit number comparison. *Journal of Experimental Psychology: Human Perception and Performance, 16*, 626–641.

4. Mehler, J., & Bever, T. G. (1967). Cognitive capacity of very young children. *Science, 158*, 141–142.

5. McGarrigle, J., & Donaldson, M. (1974). Conservation accident. *Cognition, 3*, 341–350.

6. Antell, S. E., & Keating, D. P. (1983). Perception of numerical invariance in neonates. *Child Development, 54*, 695–701.

7. Wynn, K. (1992). Addition and subtraction by human infants. *Nature, 358*, 749–750.

7a. Dumontheil, I., & Klingberg, T. (2012). Brain activity during a visuospatial working memory task predicts arithmetical performance two years later. *Cerebral Cortex, 22*, 1078–1085.

8. Gathercole, S. E., & Pickering, S. J. (2000). Working memory deficits in children with low achievements in the national curriculum at 7 years of age. *British Journal of Educational Psychology, 70*, 177–194.

9. Alloway, T. P. et al. (2009). The cognitive and behavioral characteristics of children with low working memory. *Child Development, 80*, 606–621.

10. Dehaene, S. (1997). *The number sense: How the mind creates mathematics*. New York: Oxford University Press.

11. Simon, O., et al. (2002). Topographical layout of hand, eye, calculation, and language-related areas in the human parietal lobe. *Neuron, 33*, 475–487.

12. Nieder, A., & Miller, E. K. (2004). A parieto-frontal network for visual numerical information in the monkey. *Proceedings of the National Academy of Sciences USA, 101*, 7457–7462.

13. Dumontheil, I., & Klingberg, T. (2011). Brain activity during a visuospatial working memory task predicts arithmetical performance two years later. *Cerebral Cortex, 22*, 1078–1085.

14. Sacks, O. (1987). *The man who mistook his wife for a hat*. New York: Touchstone.

15. Grafman, J., et al. (1989). Calculation abilities in a patient with virtual left hemispherectomy. *Behavioral Neurology, 2*, 183–194.

16. Dehaene, S. et al. (2004). Arithmetic and the brain. *Current Opinion in Neurobiology, 14*, 218–224.

17. Benbow, C. P., & Stanley, J. C. (1980). Sex differences in mathematical ability: Fact or artifact? *Science, 210*, 1262–1264.

18. Guiso, L. et al. (2008). Diversity: Culture, gender, and math. *Science, 320*, 1164–1165.

19. Shalev, R. S. (2004). Developmental dyscalculia. *Journal of Child Neurology, 19*, 765–771.

20. Lundberg, I., & Sterner, G. (2009). *Dyskalkyli—finns det?* Gothenburg, Sweden: National Centre for Mathematics Education at Gothenburg University.
21. Landerl, K., et al. (2009). Dyslexia and dyscalculia: Two learning disorders with different cognitive profiles. *Journal of Experimental Child Psychology, 103,* 309–324.
22. Rotzer, S., et al. (2009). Dysfunctional neural network of spatial working memory contributes to developmental dyscalculia. *Neuropsychologia, 47,* 2859–2865.
23. Price, G. R., et al. (2007). Impaired parietal magnitude processing in developmental dyscalculia. *Current Biology, 17,* R1042–R1043.
24. Cohen Kadosh, R., et al. (2007). Virtual dyscalculia induced by parietal lobe TMS impairs automatic magnitude processing. *Current Biology, 17,* 689–693.
25. Rubinstein, O., & Henik, A. (2009). Developmental dyscalcula: Heterogeneity might not mean different mechanisms. *Trends in Cognitive Science, 13,* 92–99.
26. Alarcón, M., et al. (1997). A twin study of mathematics disability. *Journal of Learning Disabilities, 30,* 617–623.
27. Shalev, R. S., et al. (2001). Developmental dyscalculia is a familial learning disability. *Journal of Learning Disabilities, 34,* 59–65.
28. Haworth, C. M., et al. (2007). Developmental origins of low mathematics performance and normal variation in twins from 7 to 9 years. *Twin Research and Human Genetics, 10,* 106–117.
29. Anderson, P., & Doyle, L. W. (2003). Neurobehavioral outcomes of school-age children born extremely low birth weight or very preterm in the 1990s. *Journal of the American Medical Association, 289,* 3264–3272.
30. Isaacs, E. B., et al. (2001). Calculation difficulties in children of very low birthweight: A neural correlate. *Brain, 124,* 1701–1707.
31. Wilson, A. J., et al. (2006). Principles underlying the design of "The Number Race," an adaptive computer game for remediation of dyscalculia. *Behavioral and Brain Functions, 2,* 19.
32. Wilson, A. J., et al. (2006). An open trial assessment of "The Number Race," an adaptive computer game for remediation of dyscalculia. *Behavioral and Brain Functions, 2,* 20.
33. Griffin, S. (2004). Number worlds: A research based mathematics program for young children. In I. Douglas, J. Sarama, & A. DiBiase (Eds.), *Engaging young children in mathematics.* Hillsdale, NJ: Erlbaum.
34. Butterworth, B., & Yeo, D. (2004). *Dyscalculia Guidance: Helping Pupils with Specific Learning Difficulties in Math.* Abingdon: Nelson Publishing Company.
35. Bor, D., et al. (2007). Savant memory for digits in a case of synaesthesia and Asperger syndrome is related to hyperactivity in the lateral prefrontal cortex. *Neurocase, 13,* 311–319.

CHAPTER 6

1. Shalev, R. S. (2004). Developmental dyscalculia. *Journal of Child Neurology, 19,* 765–771.

2. von Aster, M. G., & Shalev, R. S. (2007). Number development and developmental dyscalculia. *Development Medicine and Child Neurology, 49,* 868–873.

3. Willcutt, E. G., et al. (2010). Etiology and neuropsychology of comorbidity between RD and ADHD: The case for multipledeficit models. *Cortex, 46,* 1345–1361.

4. Lundberg, I., & Sterner, G. (2006). *Räknesvårigheter och lässvårigheter under de första skolåren—hur hänger de ihop?* Stockholm: Natur och Kultur.

5. Frith, U. (1985). Beneath the surface of developmental dyslexia. In K. E. Patterson, J. C. Marshall, & M. Coltheart (Eds.), *Surface dyslexia: Cognitive and neuropsychological studies of phonological reading.* Hillsdale, NJ: Erlbaum.

6. Puce, A., et al. (1996). Differential sensitivity of human visual cortex to faces, letterstrings, and textures: A functional magnetic resonance imaging study. *Journal of Neuroscience, 16,* 5205–5215.

7. Paulesu, E., et al. (2001). Dyslexia: Cultural diversity and biological unity. *Science, 291,* 2165–2167.

8. Dehaene, S. (2009). *Reading in the brain.* New York: Penguin.

9. Shaywitz, B. A., et al. (2002). Disruption of posterior brain systems for reading in children with developmental dyslexia. *Biological Psychiatry, 52,* 101–110.

10. Gathercole, S. E., et al. (2006). Working memory in children with reading disabilities. *Journal of Experimental Child Psychology, 93,* 265–281.

11. Silani, G., et al. (2005). Brain abnormalities underlying altered activation in dyslexia: A voxel based morphometry study. *Brain, 128,* 2453–2461.

12. Klingberg, T., et al. (2000). Microstructure of temporo-parietal white matter as a basis for reading ability: Evidence from diffusion tensor magnetic resonance imaging. *Neuron, 25,* 493–500.

13. Ramus, F., & Szenkovits, G. (2008). What phonological deficit? *Quarterly Journal of Experimental Psychology (Colchester), 61,* 129–141.

14. Kere, J., & Finer, D. (2008). *Dyslexi.* Stockholm: Karolinska Institutet University Press.

15. Galaburda, A. M., et al. (1985). Developmental dyslexia: Four consecutive patients with cortical anomalies. *Annals of Neurology, 18,* 222–233.

16. Lind, P. A., et al. (2010). Dyslexia and DCDC2: Normal variation in reading and spelling is associated with DCDC2 polymorphisms in an Australian population sample. *European Journal of Human Genetics, 18,* 668–673.

17. Lundberg, I., et al. (1988). Effects of an extensive program for stimulating phonological awareness in pre-school children. *Reading Research Quarterly*, *13*, 263–284.
18. Shaywitz, B. A., et al. (2002). Disruption of posterior brain systems for reading in children with developmental dyslexia. *Biological Psychiatry*, *52*, 101–110.
19. Maurer, U., et al. (2009). Neurophysiology in preschool improves behavioral prediction of reading ability throughout primary school. *Biological Psychiatry*, *66*, 341–348.
20. Guttorm, T. K., et al. (2005). Brain event-related potentials (ERPs) measured at birth predict later language development in children with and without familial risk for dyslexia. *Cortex*, *41*, 291–303.
21. Guttorm, T. K., et al. (2001). Event-related potentials and consonant differentiation in newborns with familial risk for dyslexia. *Journal of Learning Disabilities*, *34*, 534–544.
22. Gabrieli, J. D. (2009). Dyslexia: A new synergy between education and cognitive neuroscience. *Science*, *325*, 280–283.

CHAPTER 7

1. Beckett, C., et al. (2007). Scholastic attainment following severe early institutional deprivation: A study of children adopted from Romania. *Journal of Abnormal Child Psychology*, *35*, 1063–1073.
2. Kreppner, J. M., et al. (2007). Normality and impairment following profound early institutional deprivation: A longitudinal follow-up into early adolescence. *Developmental Psychology*, *43*, 931–946.
3. Nelson, C. A., III, et al. (2007). Cognitive recovery in socially deprived young children: The Bucharest Early Intervention Project. *Science*, *318*, 1937–1940.
4. van Praag, H., et al. (2000). Neural consequences of environmental enrichment. *Nature Reviews Neuroscience*, *1*, 191–198.
5. Markham, J. A., & Greenough, W. T. (2004). Experience-driven brain plasticity: Beyond the synapse. *Neuron Glia Biology*, *1*, 351–363.
6. Mohammed, A. H., et al. (1993). Environmental influences on the central nervous system and their implications for the aging rat. *Behavioural Brain Research*, *57*, 183–191.
7. Barnea, A., & Nottebohm, F. (1994). Seasonal recruitment of hippocampal neurons in adult free-ranging black-capped chickadees. *Proceedings of the National Academy of Sciences USA*, *91*, 11217–11221.
8. Liu, D., et al. (2000). Maternal care, hippocampal synaptogenesis and cognitive development in rats. *Nature Neuroscience*, *3*, 799–806.
9. Francis, D., et al. (1999). Nongenomic transmission across generations of maternal behavior and stress responses in the rat. *Science*, *286*, 1155–1158.
10. Weaver, I. C., et al. (2004). Epigenetic programming by maternal behaviour. *Nature Neuroscience*, *7*, 847–854.

11. McGowan, P. O., et al. (2009). Epigenetic regulation of the glucocorticoid receptor in human brain associates with childhood abuse. *Nature Neuroscience, 12,* 342–348.
12. McGeown, K. (2005). Life in Ceausescu's institutions. *BBC.* Retrieved April 2012, from http://news.bbc.co.uk/go/pr/fr/-/2/hi/europe/4630855.stm

CHAPTER 8

1. Griffith, J. D., & Hart, C. L. (2002). A summary of U.S. skydiving fatalities: 1993–1999. *Perceptual and Motor Skills, 94,* 1089–1090.
2. Leach, J., & Griffith, R. (2008). Restrictions in working memory capacity during parachuting: A possible cause of "no pull" fatalities. *Applied Cognitive Psychology, 22,* 147–157.
3. Elzinga, B. M., & Roelofs, K. (2005). Cortisol-induced impairments of working memory require acute sympathetic activation. *Behavioral Neuroscience, 119,* 98–103.
4. Lindahl, M., et al. (2005). Test performance and self-esteem in relation to experienced stress in Swedish sixth and ninth graders—saliva cortisol levels and psychological reactions to demands. *Acta Paediatrica, 94,* 489–495.
5. Roozendaal, B., et al. (2009). Stress, memory and the amygdale. *Nature Reviews Neuroscience, 10,* 423–433.
6. Arnsten, A. F. (2009). Stress signalling pathways that impair prefrontal cortex structure and function. *Nature Reviews Neuroscience, 10,* 410–422.
7. Steele, C. M., & Aronson, J. (1995). Stereotype threat and the intellectual test performance of African Americans. *Journal of Personality and Social Psychology, 69,* 797–811.
8. Schmader, T., & Johns, M. (2003). Converging evidence that stereotype threat reduces working memory capacity. *Journal of Personality and Social Psychology, 85,* 440–452.
9. Radley, J. J., et al. (2005). Reversibility of apical dendritic retraction in the rat medial prefrontal cortex following repeated stress. *Experimental Neurology, 196,* 199–203.
10. Liston, C., et al. (2009). Psychosocial stress reversibly disrupts prefrontal processing and attentional control. *Proceedings of the National Academy of Sciences USA, 106,* 912–917.
11. Evans, G. W., & Schamberg, M. A. (2009). Childhood poverty, chronic stress, and adult working memory, *Proceedings of the National Academy of Sciences USA, 106,* 6545–6549.
12. Gustafsson, J-E., et al. (2010). *School, learning and mental health.* Stockholm: Kungliga Vetenskapsakademien.

CHAPTER 9

1. Owen, A. M., et al. (2010.). Putting brain training to the test. *Nature, 465*(7299), 775–778.

2. Scruggs, T. E., & Mastropieri, M. A. (1991). Classroom applications of mnemonic instruction: Acquisition, maintenance, and generalization. *Exceptional Children, 58*, 219–229.

3. Scruggs, T. E., et al. (1985). Vocabulary acquisition by mentally retarded students under direct and mnemonic instruction. *American Journal of Mental Deficiency, 89*, 546–551.

4. Maguire, E. A., et al. (2003). Routes to remembering: The brains behind superior memory. *Nature Neuroscience, 6*, 90–95.

5. Klingberg, T., et al. (2005). Computerized training of working memory in children with ADHD—a randomized, controlled trial. *Journal of the American Academy of Child and Adolescent Psychiatry, 44*, 177–186.

6. Klingberg, T. (2010). Training and plasticity of working memory. *Trends in Cognitive Science, 14*, 317–324.

7. Thorell, L. B., et al. (2009). Training and transfer effects of executive functions in preschool children. *Developmental Science, 12*, 106–113.

8. Holmes, J., et al. (2009). Adaptive training leads to sustained enhancement of poor working memory in children. *Developmental Science, 12*, F9–F15.

9. Mezzacappa, E., & Buckner, J. C. (2010). Working memory training for children with attention problems or hyperactivity: A school-based pilot study. *School Mental Health*, doi 10.1007/ s12310-010-9030-9.

10. Beck, S. J., et al. (2010). A controlled trial of working memory training for children and adolescents with ADHD. *Journal of Clinical and Adolescent Psychology, 39*, 825–836.

11. Green et al. (in press). Will working memory training generalize to improve off-task behavior in children with attention-deficit/hyperactivity disorder? *Journal of Neurotherapeutics*.

12. Kane, M. J., et al. (2007). For whom the mind wanders, and when: An experience-sampling study of working memory and executive control in daily life. *Psychological Science, 18*, 614–621.

13. Olesen, P., et al. (2004). Increased prefrontal and parietal brain activity after training of working memory. *Nature Neuroscience, 7*, 75–79.

14. Dahlin, E., et al. (2008). Transfer of learning after updating training mediated by the striatum. *Science, 320*, 1510–1512.

15. McNab, F., et al. (2009). Changes in cortical dopamine D1 receptor binding associated with cognitive training. *Science, 323*, 800–802.

16. Dahlin, E., et al. (2008). Plasticity of executive functioning in young and older adults: Immediate training gains, transfer, and long-term maintenance. *Psychology and Aging, 23*, 720–730.

17. Jaeggi, S. M., et al. (2008). Improving fluid intelligence with training on working memory. *Proceedings of the National Academy of Sciences USA, 105*, 6829–6833.

18. Bergman Nutley, S., et al. (2011). Gains in fluid intelligence after training non-verbal reasoning in 4-year-old children: A controlled, randomized study. *Development Science, 14*(3), 591–601.

19. Diamond, A., et al. (2007). Preschool program improves cognitive control. *Science, 318,* 1387–1388.
20. Schellenberg, E. G. (2004). Music lessons enhance IQ. *Psychological Science, 15,* 511–514.
21. Bergman Nutley, S. et al. (2011). Gains in fluid intelligence after training non-verbal reasoning in 4-year-old children: A controlled, randomized study. *Development Science, 14*(3), 591–601.
22. Green, C. S., & Bavelier, D. (2003). Action video game modifies visual selective attention. *Nature, 423,* 534–537.
23. Boot, W. R., et al. (2008). The effects of video game playing on attention, memory, and executive control. *Acta Psychologica, 129,* 387–398.

CHAPTER 10

1. Colcombe, S. J., et al. (2004). Cardiovascular fitness, cortical plasticity, and aging. *Proceedings of the National Academy of Sciences USA, 101,* 3316–3321.
2. Colcombe, S. J., et al. (2006). Aerobic exercise training increases brain volume in aging humans. *The Journal of Gerontology. Series A, Biological Sciences and Medical Sciences, 61,* 1166–1170.
3. Pereira, A. C., et al. (2007). An in vivo correlate of exercise-induced neurogenesis in the adult dentate gyrus, *Proceedings of the National Academy of Sciences USA, 104,* 5638–5643.
4. Hillman, C. H., et al. (2008). Be smart, exercise your heart: Exercise effects on brain and cognition. *Nature Reviews Neuroscience, 9,* 58–65.
5. Erickson, K. I., et al. (2010). Brain-derived neurotrophic factor is associated with age-related decline in hippocampal volume. *Journal of Neuroscience, 30,* 5368–5375.
6. Ratey, J. (2008). *Spark.* Boston, MA: Little, Brown.
7. Ferris, L. T., et al. (2007). The effect of acute exercise on serum brain-derived neurotrophic factor levels and cognitive function. *Medicine and Science in Sports and Exercise, 39,* 728–734.
8. Sibley, B. A., & Etnier, J. L. (2003). The relationship between physical activity and cognition in children: A meta-analysis. *Pediactric Exercise Science, 15,* 243–256.
9. Richardson, A. J., & Montgomery, P. (2005). The Oxford-Durham study: A randomized, controlled trial of dietary supplementation with fatty acids in children with developmental coordination disorder. *Pediatrics, 115,* 1360–1366.
10. Voigt, R. G., et al. (2001). A randomized, double-blind, placebo-controlled trial of docosahexaenoic acid supplementation in children with attention-deficit/hyperactivity disorder. *Journal of Pediatrics, 139,* 189–196.
11. Hirayama, S., et al. (2004). Effect of docosahexaenoic acid-containing food administration on symptoms of attention-deficit/hyperactivity

disorder—a placebo-controlled double-blind study. *European Journal of Clinical Nutrition, 58,* 467–473.

12. Eppig, C., et al. (2010). Parasite prevalence and the worldwide distribution of cognitive ability, *Proceedings in Biological Sciences, 277,* 3801–3808.

CHAPTER 11

1. Meltzoff, A. N., et al. (2009). Foundations for a new science of learning. *Science, 325,* 284–288.
2. Stephenson, N. (1996). *The diamond age—or a young lady's illustrated primer.* New York: Bantam Books.
3. Bringuier, J-C. (1989). *Conversations with Jean Piaget.* Chicago, IL: University of Chicago Press.
4. Brockman, J. (2010). *This will change everything—ideas that will shape the future.* San Francisco, CA: Harper Collins.

BIBLIOGRAPHY

Alarcón, M., DeFries, J. C., Light, J. G., & Pennington, B. F. (1997). A twin study of mathematics disability. *Journal of Learning Disabilities, 30,* 617–623.

Alexander, D. M., Williams, L. M., Gatt, J. M., Dobson-Stone, C., Kuan, S. A., Todd, E. G.,... Gordon, E. (2007). The contribution of apolipoprotein E alleles on cognitive performance and dynamic neural activity over six decades. *Biological Psychology, 75,* 229–238.

Alloway, T. P., Gathercole, S. E., Kirkwood, H., & Elliott, J. (2009). The cognitive and behavioral characteristics of children with low working memory. *Child Development, 80,* 606–621.

Anderson, P., & Doyle, L.W. (2003). "Neurobehavioral outcomes of school-age children born extremely low birth weight or very preterm in the 1990s. *JAMA,* 289, 3264–3272.

Antell, S. E., & Keating, D. P. (1983). Perception of numerical invariance in neonates. *Child Development, 54,* 695–701.

Arnsten, A. F. (2009). Stress signalling pathways that impair prefrontal cortex structure and function. *Nature Reviews Neuroscience, 10,* 410–422.

von Aster, M. G., & Shalev, R. S. (2007). Number development and developmental dyscalculia. *Development Medicine and Child Neurology, 49,* 868–873.

Bainbridge, D. (2009). *Teenagers—a natural history.* Toronto, ON: Greystone Books.

Baker-Ward, L., & Ornstein, P. A. (1988). Age differences in visualspatial memory performance: Do children really out-perform adults when playing concentrations? *Bulletin of the Psychonomic Society, 26,* 331–332.

Barnea, A., & Nottebohm, F. (1994). Seasonal recruitment of hippocampal neurons in adult free-ranging black-capped chickadees. *Proceedings of the National Academy of Sciences USA, 91,* 11217–11221.

BBC. (2008). *How does your memory work?* [television program]. London: BBC.

Beck, S. J., Hanson, C. A., Puffenberger, S. S., Benninger, K. L., & Benninger, W. B. (2010). A controlled trial of working memory training for children and adolescents with ADHD. *Journal of Clinical and Adolescent Psychology, 39*, 825–836.

Beckett, C., Maughan, B., Rutter, M., Castle, J., Colvert, E., Groothues, C.,...Sonuga-Barke. E. J. (2007). Scholastic attainment following severe early institutional deprivation: A study of children adopted from Romania. *Journal of Abnormal Child Psychology, 35*, 1063–1073.

Benbow, C. P., & Stanley, J. C. (1980). Sex differences in mathematical ability: Fact or artifact? *Science, 210*, 1262–1264.

Bergman Nutley, S., Söderqvist, S., Bryde, S., Thorell, L. B., Humphreys, K., & Klingberg, T. (2011). Gains in fluid intelligence after training non-verbal reasoning in 4-year-old children: A controlled, randomized study. *Development Science, 14*(3), 591–601.

Boot, W. R., Kramer, A. F., Simons, D. J., Fabiani, M., & Gratton, G. (2008). The effects of video game playing on attention, memory, and executive control. *Acta Psychologica, 129*, 387–398.

Bor, D., Billington, J., & Baron-Cohen, S. (2007). Savant memory for digits in a case of synaesthesia and Asperger syndrome is related to hyperactivity in the lateral prefrontal cortex. *Neurocase, 13*, 311–319.

Brandt, K. R., Gardiner, J. M., Vargha-Khadem, F., Baddeley, A. D., & Mishkin, M. (2008). Impairment of recollection but not familiarity in a case of developmental amnesia. *Neurocase, 15*, 60–65.

Bringuier, J-C. (1989). *Conversations with Jean Piaget*. Chicago, IL: University of Chicago Press.

Brockman, J. (2010). *This will change everything—ideas that will shape the future*. San Francisco, CA: Harper Collins.

Brown, A. L., & Scott, M. S. (1971). Recognition memory for pictures in preschool children. *Journal of Experimental Child Psychology, 11*, 401–412.

Butterworth, B., & Yeo, D. (2010). *Dyscalulia: Helping children with specific mathematic disabilities*. Stockholm: Natur & Kultur.

Castellanos, F. X., Lee, P. P., Sharp, W., Jeffries, N. O., Greenstein, D. K., Clasen, L. S.,...Rapoport, J. L. (2002). Developmental trajectories of brain volume abnormalities in children and adolescents with attention deficit/hyperactivity disorder. *Journal of the American Medical Association, 288*, 1740–1748.

Cauffman, E., Shulman, E. P., Steinberg, L., Claus, E., Banich, M. T., Graham, S., & Woolard, J. (2010). Age differences in affective decision making as indexed by performance on the Iowa Gambling Task. *Developmental Psychology, 46*, 193–207.

Chugani, H. T., Phelps, M. E., & Maziotta, J. C. (1987). Positron emission tomography study of human brain functional development. *Annals of Neurology, 22*, 487–497.

Cohen, J. R., Asarnow, R. F., Sabb, F. W., Bilder, R. M., Bookheimer, S. Y., Knowlton, B. J., & Poldrack, R. A. (2010). A unique adolescent response to reward prediction errors. *Nature Neuroscience, 13*, 669–671.

Cohen Kadosh, R., Cohen Kadosh, K., Schuhmann, T., Kaas, A., Goebel, R., Henik, A., & Sack, A. T. (2007). Virtual dyscalculia induced by parietal lobe TMS impairs automatic magnitude processing. *Current Biology, 17,* 689–693.

Colombe, S. J., Kramer, A. F., Erickson, K. I., Scalf, P., McAuley, E., Cohen, N. J., . . . Elavsky, S. (2004). Cardiovascular fitness, cortical plasticity, and aging. *Proceedings of the National Academy of Sciences USA, 101,* 3316–3321.

Colombe, S. J., Erickson, K. I., Scalf, P. E., Kim, J. S., Prakash, R., McAuley, E., . . . Kramer, A. F. (2006). Aerobic exercise training increases brain volume in aging humans. *The Journal of Gerontology. Series A, Biological Sciences and Medical Sciences, 61,* 1166–1170.

Dahlin, E., Neely, A. S., Larsson, A., Bäckman, L., & Nyberg, L. (2008). Transfer of learning after updating training mediated by the striatum. *Science, 320,* 1510–1512.

Dahlin, E., Nyberg, L., Bäckman, L., & Neely, A. S. (2008). Plasticity of executive functioning in young and older adults: Immediate training gains, transfer, and long-term maintenance. *Psychology and Aging, 23,* 720–730.

Dehaene, S. (1997). *The number sense. How the mind creates mathematics.* New York: Oxford University Press.

Dehaene, S. (2009). *Reading in the brain.* New York: Penguin Group.

Dehaene, S., Bossini, S., & Giraux, P. (1993). The mental representation of parity and numerical magnitude. *Journal of Experimental Psychology: General, 122,* 371–396.

Dehaene, S., Dupoux, E., & Mehler, J. (1990). Is numerical comparison digital? Analogical and symbolic effects in two-digit number comparison. *Journal of Experimental Psychology. Human Perception and Performance, 16,* 626–641.

Dehaene, S., Molko, N., Cohen, L., & Wilson, A. J. (2004). Arithmetic and the brain. *Current Opinion in Neurobiology, 14,* 218–224.

Diamond, A., Barnett, W. S., Thomas, J., & Munro, S. (2007). Preschool program improves cognitive control. *Science, 318,* 1387–1388.

Elzinga, B. M., & Roelofs, K. (2005). Cortisol-induced impairments of working memory require acute sympathetic activation. *Behavioral Neuroscience, 119,* 98–103.

Eppig, C., Fincher, C. L., & Thornhill, R. (2010). Parasite prevalence and the worldwide distribution of cognitive ability. *Proceeding in Biological Sciences, 277,* 3801–3808.

Erickson, K. I,. Prakash, R. S., Voss, M. W., Chaddock, L., Heo, S., McLaren, M., . . . Kramer, A. F. (2010). Brain-derived neurotrophic factor is associated with age-related decline in hippocampal volume. *Journal of Neuroscience, 30,* 5368–5375.

Evans, G. W., & Schamberg, M. A. (2009). Childhood poverty, chronic stress, and adult working memory. *Proceedings of the National Academy of Sciences USA, 106,* 6545–6549.

Ferris, L. T., Williams, J. S., & Shen, C. L. (2007). The effect of acute exercise on serum brain-derived neurotrophic factor levels and cognitive function. *Medicine and Science in Sports and Exercise, 39,* 728–734.

Francis, D., Diorio, J., Liu, D., & Meaney, M. J. (1999). Nongenomic transmission across generations of maternal behavior and stress responses in the rat. *Science, 286,* 1155–1158.

Friedman, N. P., Miyake, A., Young, S. E., Defries, J. C., Corley, R. P., & Hewitt, J. K. (2008). Individual differences in executive functions are almost entirely genetic in origin. *Journal of Experimental Psychology: General, 137,* 201–225.

Frith, U. (1985). Beneath the surface of developmental dyslexia. In K. E. Patterson, J. C. Marshall, & M. Coltheart (Eds.), *Surface dyslexia: Cognitive and neuropsychological studies of phonological reading.* Hillsdale, NJ: Erlbaum.

Gabrieli, J. D. (2009). Dyslexia: A new synergy between education and cognitive neuroscience. *Science, 325,* 280–283.

Galaburda, A. M., Sherman, G. F., Rosen, G. D., Aboitiz, F., & Geschwind, N. (1985). Developmental dyslexia: Four consecutive patients with cortical anomalies. *Annals of Neurology, 18,* 222–233.

Gathercole S. E., & Alloway, T. P. (2008). *Working memory and learning: A practical guide for teachers.* Thousand Oaks, CA: Sage Publications.

Gathercole, S. E., Alloway, T. P., Willis, C., & Adams, A. M. (2006). Working memory in children with reading disabilities. *Journal of Experimental Child Psychology, 93,* 265–281.

Gathercole, S. E., & Pickering, S. J. (2000). Working memory deficits in children with low achievements in the national curriculum at 7 years of age. *British Journal of Educational Psychology, 70,* 177–194.

Giedd, J. N., Blumenthal, J., Jeffries, N. O., Castellanos, F. X., Liu, H., Zijdenbos, A.,...Rapoport, J. L. (1999). Brain development during childhood and adolescence: A longitudinal MRI study. *Nature Neuroscience, 2,* 861–863.

Goswami, U. (2008). *Cognitive development—the learning brain.* East Sussex, UK: Psychology Press.

Gould, E., Reeves, A. J., Fallah, M., Tanapat, P., Gross, C. G., & Fuchs, E. (1999). Hippocampal neurogenesis in adult Old World primate. *Proceedings of the National Academy of Sciences USA, 96,* 5263–5267.

Grafman, J., Kampen, D., Rosenberg, J., et al. (1989). Calculation abilities in a patient with virtual left hemispherectomy. *Behavioral Neurology, 2,* 183–194.

Green, C. S., & Bavelier, D. (2003). Action video game modifies visual selective attention. *Nature, 423,* 534–537.

Green et al. (in press). Will working memory training generalize to improve off-task behavior in children with attention-deficit/hyperactivity disorder? *Journal of Neurotherapeutics.*

Griffin, S. (2004). Number worlds: A research based mathematics program for young children. In I. Douglas, J. Sarama, & A. DiBiase (Eds.), *Engaging young children in mathematics*. Hillsdale, NJ: Erlbaum.

Griffith, J. D., & Hart, C. L. (2002). A summary of U.S. skydiving fatalities: 1993–1999. *Perceptual and Motor Skills, 94*, 1089–1090.

Guiso, L., Monte, F., Sapienza, P., & Zingales, L. (2008). Diversity. Culture, gender, and math. *Science, 320*, 1164–1165.

Gulya, M., Rossi-George, A., Hartshorn, K., Vieira, A., Rovee-Collier, C., Johnson, M. K., & Chalfonte, B. L. (2002). The development of explicit memory for basic perceptual feature. *Journal of Experimental Child Psychology, 81*, 276–297.

Gustafsson, J-E., Westling Allodi. M., Eriksson, C., Fischbein, S., Granlund, M., Gustafsson, P., et al. (2010). *School, learning and mental health*. Stockholm: Kungliga Vetenskapsakademien.

Guttorm, T. K., Leppänen, P. H., Poikkeus, A. M., Eklund, K. M., Lyytinen, P., & Lyytinen, H. (2005). Brain event-related potentials (ERPs) measured at birth predict later language development in children with and without familial risk for dyslexia. *Cortex, 41*, 291–303.

Guttorm, T. K., Leppänen, P. H., Richardson, U., & Lyytinen, H. (2001). Event-related potentials and consonant differentiation in newborns with familial risk for dyslexia. *Journal of Learning Disabilities, 34*, 534–544.

Haworth, C. M., Kovas, Y., Petrill, S. A., & Plomin, R. (2007). Developmental origins of low mathematics performance and normal variation in twins from 7 to 9 years. *Twin Research and Human Genetics, 10*, 106–117.

Hillman, C. H., Erickson, K. I., & Kramer, A. F. (2008). Be smart, exercise your heart: Exercise effects on brain and cognition. *Nature Reviews Neuroscience, 9*, 58–65.

Hirayama, S., Hamazaki, T., & Terasawa, K. (2004). Effect of docosahexaenoic acid-containing food administration on symptoms of attention-deficit/ hyperactivity disorder—a placebo-controlled double-blind study. *European Journal of Clinical Nutrition, 58*, 467–473.

Holmes, J., Gathercole, S. E., & Dunning, D. L. (2009). Adaptive training leads to sustained enhancement of poor working memory in children. *Developmental Science, 12*, F9–F15.

Hubacek, J. A., Pitha, J., Skodová, Z., Adámková, V., Lánská, V., & Poledne, R. (2001). A possible role of apolipoprotein E polymorphism in predisposition to higher education. *Neuropsychobiology, 43*, 200–203.

Isaacs, E. B., Edmonds, C. J., Lucas, A., & Gadian, D. G. (2001). Calculation difficulties in children of very low birthweight: A neural correlate. *Brain, 124*, 1701–1707.

Jaeggi, S. M., Buschkuehl, M., Jonides, J., & Perrig, W. J. (2008). Improving fluid intelligence with training on working memory. *Proceedings of the National Academy of Sciences USA, 105*, 6829–6833.

Kane, M. J., Brown, L. H., McVay, J. C., Silvia, P. J., Myin-Germeys, I., & Kwapil, T. R. (2007). For whom the mind wanders, and when: An experience-sampling study of working memory and executive control in daily life. *Psychological Science, 18*, 614–621.

Kelly, K., & Ramundo, P. (2006). *You mean I'm not lazy, stupid or crazy?! A self-help book for adults with attention deficit disorder.* New York: Simon & Schuster.

Kere, J., & Finer, D. (2008). *Dyslexi.* Stockhom: Karolinska Institutet University Press.

Klingberg, T. (2006). Development of a superior frontal-intraparietal network for visuo-spatial working memory. *Neuropsychologia, 44,* 2171–2177.

Klingberg, T. (2010). Training and plasticity of working memory. *Trends in Cognitive Science, 14,* 317–324.

Klingberg, T., Fernell, E., Olesen, P. J., Johnson, M., Gustafsson, P., Dahlström, K.,...Westerberg, H. (2005). Computerized training of working memory in children with ADHD—a randomized, controlled trial. *Journal of the American Academy of Child and Adolescent Psychiatry, 44,* 177–186.

Klingberg, T., Hedehus, M., Temple, E., Salz, T., Gabrieli, J. D., Moseley, M. E., & Poldrack, R. A. (2000). Microstructure of temporoparietal white matter as a basis for reading ability: Evidence from diffusion tensor magnetic resonance imagines. *Neuron, 25,* 493–500.

Kreppner, J. M., Rutter, M., Beckett, C., Castle, J., Colvert, E., Groothues, C.,...Sonuga-Barke, E. J. (2007). Normality and impairment following profound early institutional deprivation: A longitudinal follow-up into early adolescence. *Developmental Psychology, 43,* 931–946.

Landauer, T. K., & Bjork, R. A. (1978). Optimum rehearsal patterns and name learning. In M. M. Gruneberg, P. E. Morris, & R. N. Sykes (Eds.), *Practical aspects of memory.* San Diego, CA: Academic Press.

Landerl, K., Fussenegger, B., Moll, K., & Willburger, E. (2009). Dyslexia and dyscalculia: Two learning disorders with different cognitive profiles. *Journal of Experimental Child Psychology, 103,* 309–324.

Leach, J., & Griffith, R. (2008). Restrictions in working memory capacity during parachuting: A possible cause of "no pull" fatalities. *Applied Cognitive Psychology, 22,* 147–157.

van Leijonhorst, L., Zanolie, K., van Meel, C. S., Westenberg, P. M., Rombouts, S. A., & Crone, E. A. (2010). What motivates the adolescent? Brain regions mediating reward sensitivity across adolescence. *Cerebral Cortex, 20,* 61–69.

Lind, P. A., Luciano, M., Wright, M. J., Montgomery, G. W., Martin, N. G., & Bates, T. C. (2010). Dyslexia and DCDC2: Normal variation in reading and spelling is associated with DCDC2 polymorphisms in an Australian population sample. *European Journal of Human Genetics, 18,* 668–673.

Lindahl, M., Theorell, T., & Lindblad, F. (2005). Test performance and self-esteem in relation to experienced stress in Swedish sixth and ninth graders-saliva cortisol levels and psychological reactions to demands. *Acta Paediatrica, 94,* 489–495.

Liston, C., McEwen, B. S., & Casey, B. J. (2009). Psychosocial stress reversibly disrupts prefrontal processing and attentional control. *Proceedings of the National Academy of Sciences USA, 106,* 912–917.

Liu, D., Diorio, J., Day, J. C., Francis, D. D., & Meaney, M. J. (2000). Maternal care, hippocampal synaptogenesis and cognitive development in rats. *Nature Neuroscience, 3,* 799–806.

Luciano, M., Wright, M., Smith, G. A., Geffen, G. M., Geffen, L. B., & Martin, N. G. (2001). Genetic covariance among measures of information processing speed, working memory, and IQ. *Behavioral Genetics, 31,* 581–592.

Lundberg, I., & Sterner, G. (2006). *Räknesvårigheter och lässvårigheter under de första skolåren—hur hänger de ihop?* Stockholm: Natur & Kultur.

Lundberg, I., & Sterner, G. (2009). *Dyskalkyli—finns det?* Gothenburg, Sweden: National Centre for Mathematics Education at Gothenburg University.

Lundberg, I., Frost, J., & Petersen, O-P. (1988). Effects of an extensive program for stimulating phonological awareness in pre-school children. *Reading Research Quarterly, 13,* 263–284.

Maddrey, A. M., Bergeron, J. A., Lombardo, E. R., McDonald, N. K., Mulne, A. F., Barenberg, P. D., & Bowers, D. C. (2005). Neuropsychological performance and quality of life of 10 year survivors of childhood medulloblastoma. *Journal of Neurooncology, 72,* 245–253.

Maguire, E. A., Valentine, E. R., Wilding, J. M., & Kapur, N. (2003). Routes to remembering: the brains behind superior memory. *Nature Neuroscience, 6,* 90–95.

Markham, J. A., & Greenough, W. T. (2004). Experience-driven brain plasticity: beyond the synapse. *Neuron Glia Biology, 1,* 351–363.

Maurer, U., Bucher, K., Brem, S., Benz, R., Kranz, F., Schulz, E., . . . Brandeis, D. (2009). Neurophysiology in preschool improves behavioural prediction of reading ability throughout primary school. *Biological Psychiatry, 66,* 341–348.

McGarrigle, J., & Donaldson, M. (1974 ed.). Conservation accidents. *Cognition, 3,* 341–350.

McGeown, K. (2005). Life in Ceausescu's institutions. *BBC.* Retrieved April 2012, from http://news.bbc.co.uk/go/pr/fr/-/2/hi/europe/4630855.stm

McGowan, P. O., Sasaki, A., D'Alessio, A. C., Dymov, S., Labonté, B., Szyf, M., . . . Meaney, M. J. (2009). Epigenetic regulation of the glucocorticoid receptor in human brain associates with childhood abuse. *Nature Neuroscience, 12,* 342–348.

McNab, F., Varrone, A., Farde, L., Jucaite, A., Bystritsky, P., Forssberg, H., & Klingberg, T. (2009). Changes in cortical dopamine D1 receptor binding associated with cognitive training. *Science, 323*, 800–802.

Mehler, J., & Bever, T. G. (1967). Cognitive capacity of very young children. *Science, 158*, 141–142.

Meltzoff, A. N., Kuhl, P. K., Movellan, J., & Sejnowski, T. J. (2009). Foundations for a new science of learning. *Science, 325*, 284–288.

Mezzacappa, E., & Buckner, J. C. (2010). Working memory training for children with attention problems or hyperactivity: A school-based pilot study. *School Mental Health*, doi: 10.1007/ s12310-010-9030-9.

Mohammed, A. H., Henriksson, B. G., Söderström, S., Ebendal, T., Olsson, T., & Seckl, J. R. (1993). Environmental influences on the central nervous system and their implications for the aging rat. *Behavioural Brain Research, 57*, 183–191.

Nagy, Z., Westerberg, H., & Klingberg, T. (2004). Regional maturation of white matter during childhood and development of function. *Journal of Cognitive Neuroscience, 16*, 1227–1233.

Nelson, C. A., III, Zeanah, C. H., Fox, N. A., Marshall, P. J., Smyke, A. T., & Guthrie D. (2007). Cognitive recovery in socially deprived young children: The Bucharest Early Intervention Project. *Science, 318*, 1937–1940.

Nieder, A., & Miller, E. K. (2004). A parieto-frontal network for visual numerical information in the monkey. *Proceedings of the National Academy of Sciences USA, 101*, 7457–7462.

Nilsson, B. B. (2007). *Nej, jag är inte dum . . . jag har bara lite otur när jag tänker.* Burgsvik, Sweden: Valar Press.

Obituary. (2008 December 20). *The Economist*, p. 134.

Olesen, P., Westerberg, H., & Klingberg, T. (2004). Increased prefrontal and parietal brain activity after training of working memory. *Nature Neuroscience, 7*, 75–79.

Owen, A. M., Hampshire, A., Grahn, J. A., Stenton, R., Dajani, S., Burns, A. S., . . . Ballard, C. G. (2010). Putting brain training to the test. *Nature, 465*(7299). 775–778.

Paulesu, E., Démonet, J. F., Fazio, F., McCrory, E., Chanoine, V., Brunswick, N., Cappa, S. F., . . . Frith, U. (2001). Dyslexia: Cultural diversity and biological unity. *Science, 291*, 2165–2167.

Pereira, A. C., Huddleston, D. E., Brickman, A. M., Sosunov, A. A., Hen, R., McKhann, G. M., . . . Small, S. A. (2007). An in vivo correlate of exercise-induced neurogenesis in the adult dentate gyrus. *Proceedings of the National Academy of Sciences USA, 104*, 5638–5643.

van Praag, H., Kemperman, G., & Gage, F. H. (2000). Neural consequences of environmental enrichment. *Nature Reviews Neuroscience, 1*, 191–198.

Price, G. R., Holloway, I., Räsänen, P., Vesterinen, M., & Ansari, D. (2007). Impaired parietal magnitude processing in developmental dyscalculia. *Current Biology, 17*, R1042–R1043.

Puce, A., Allison, T., Asgari, M., Gore, J. C., & McCarthy, G. (1996). Differential sensitivity of human visual cortex to faces, letterstrings, and textures: A functional magnetic resonance imaging study. *Journal of Neuroscience, 16,* 5205–5215.

Radley, J. J., Rocher, A. B., Janssen, W. G., Hof, P. R., McEwen, B. S., & Morrison, J. H. (2005). Reversibility of apical dendritic retraction in the rat medial prefrontal cortex following repeated stress. *Experimental Neurology, 196,* 199–203.

Ramus, F., & Szenkovits, G. (2008). What phonological deficit? *The Quarterly Journal of Experimental Psychology (Colchester), 61,* 129–141.

Ratey, J. (2008). *Spark.* Boston, MA: Little, Brown.

Richardson, A. J., & Montgomery, P. (2005). The Oxford-Durham study: A randomized, controlled trial of dietary supplementation with fatty acids in children with developmental coordination disorder. *Pediatrics, 115,* 1360–1366.

Richmond, J., & Nelson, C. A. (2007). Accounting for change in declarative memory: A cognitive neuroscience perspective. *Developmental Review, 27,* 349–373.

Roozendaal, B., McEwen, B. S., & Chattarji, S. (2009). Stress, memory and the amygdale. *Nature Reviews Neuroscience, 10,* 423–433.

Rotzer, S., Loenneker, T., Kucian, K., Martin, E., Klaver, P., & von Aster, M. (2009). Dysfunctional neural network of spatial working memory contributes to developmental dyscalculia. *Neuropsychologia, 47,* 2859–2865.

Rubinstein, O., & Henik, A. (2009). Developmental dyscalculia: Heterogeneity might not mean different mechanisms. *Trends in Cognitive Science, 13,* 92–99.

Sacks, O. (1987). *The man who mistook his wife for a hat.* New York: Touchstone.

Schellenberg, E. G. (2004). Music lessons enhance IQ. *Psychological Science, 15,* 511–514.

Schmader, T., & Johns, M. (2003). Converging evidence that stereotype threat reduces working memory capacity. *Journal of Personality and Social Psychology, 85,* 440–452.

Scruggs, T. E., & Mastropieri, M. A. (1991). Classroom applications of mnemonic instruction: Acquisition, maintenance, and generalization. *Exceptional Children, 58,* 219–229.

Scruggs, T. E., Mastropieri, M. A., & Levin, J. R. (1985). Vocabulary acquisition by mentally retarded students under direct and mnemonic instruction. *American Journal of Mental Deficiency, 89,* 546–551.

Shalev, R. S. (2004). Developmental dyscalculia. *Journal of Child Neurology, 19,* 765–771.

Shalev, R. S., Manor, O., Kerem, B., Ayali, M., Badichi, N., Friedlander, Y., & Gross-Tsur, V. (2001). Developmental dyscalculia is a familial learning disability. *Journal of Learning Disabilities, 34,* 59–65.

Shaw, P., Eckstrand, K., Sharp, W., Blumenthal, J., Lerch, J. P., Greenstein, D., ... Rapoport, J. L. (2007). Attention-deficit/hyperactivity disorder is characterized by a delay in cortical maturation. *Proceedings of the National Academy of Sciences USA, 104*(49), 19649–19654.

Shaw, P., Kabani, N. J., Lerch, J. P., Eckstrand, K., Lenroot, R., Gogtay, N., ... Wise, S. P. (2008). Neurodevelopmental trajectories of the human cerebral cortex. *Journal of Neuroscience, 28,* 3586–3594.

Shaywitz, B. A., Shaywitz, S. E., Pugh, K. R., Mencl, W. E., Fulbright, R. K., Skudlarski, P., ... Gore, J. C. (2002). Disruption of posterior brain systems for reading in children with developmental dyslexia. *Biological Psychiatry, 52,* 101–110.

Sibley, B. A., & Etnier, J. L. (2003). The relationship between physical activity and cognition in children: A meta-analysis. *Pediactric Exercise Science, 15,* 243–256.

Silani, G., Frith, U., Demonet, J. F., Fazio, F., Perani, D., Price, C., ... Paulesu, E. (2005). Brain abnormalities underlying altered activation in dyslexia: A voxel based morphometry study. *Brain, 128,* 2453–2461.

Simon, O., Mangin, J. F., Cohen, L., Le Bihan, D., & Dehaene, S. (2002). Topographical layout of hand, eye, calculation, and language-related areas in the human parietal lobe. *Neuron, 33,* 475–487.

Somerville, L. H., & Casey, B. J. (2010). Developmental neurobiology of cognitive control and motivational systems. *Current Opinion in Neurobiology, 20,* 236–241.

Steele, C. M., & Aronson, J. (1995). Stereotype threat and the intellectual test performance of African Americans. *Journal of Personality and Social Psychology, 69,* 797–811.

Stephenson, N. (1996). *The diamond age—or a young lady's illustrated primer.* New York: Bantam Books.

Söderqvist, S., McNab, F., Peyrard-Janvid, M., Matsson, H., Humphreys, K., Kere, J., & Klingberg, T. (2010). The SNAP25 gene is linked to working memory capacity and maturation of the posterior cingulate cortex during childhood. *Biological Psychiatry, 68,* 1120–1125.

Tammet, D. (2008). *Born on a blue day.* New York: Free Press.

Tang, Y. P., Shimizu, E., Dube, G. R., Rampon, C., Kerchner, G. A., Zhuo, M., ... Tsien, J. Z. (1999). Genetic enhancement of learning and memory in mice. *Nature, 401,* 63–69.

Teach ADHD. (2010). Retrieved April 2012, from http://research.about-kidshealth.ca/teachadhd/about

Thorell, L. B., Lindqvist, S., Bergman Nutley, S., Bohlin, G., & Klingberg, T. (2009). Training and transfer effects of executive functions in preschool children. *Developmental Science, 12,* 106–113.

Weaver, I. C., Cervoni, N., Champagne, F. A., D'Alessio, A. C., Sharma, S., Seckl, J. R., ... Meaney, M. J. (2004). Epigenetic programming by maternal behaviour. *Nature Neuroscience, 7,* 847–854.

Willcutt, E. G., Betjemann, R. S., McGrath, L. M., Chhabildas, N. A., Olson, R. K., DeFries, J. C., & Pennington, B. F. (2010). Etiology and neuropsychology of comorbidity between RD and ADHD: The case for multiple-deficit models. *Cortex, 46,* 1345–1361.

Wilson, A. J., Dehaene, S., Pinel, P., Revkin, S. K., Cohen, L., & Cohen, D. (2006). Principles underlying the design of "The Number Race," an adaptive computer game for remediation of dyscalculia. *Behavioral and Brain Functions, 2,* 19.

Wilson, A. J., Revkin, S. K., Cohen, D., Cohen, L., & Dehaene, S. (2006). An open trial assessment of "The Number Race," an adaptive computer game for remediation of dyscalculia. *Behavioral and Brain Function, 2,* 20.

Voigt, R. G., Llorente, A. M., Jensen, C. L., Fraley, J. K., Berretta, M. C., & Heird, W. C. (2001). A randomized, double-blind, placebo-controlled trial of docosahexaenoic acid supplementation in children with attention deficit/hyperactivity disorder. *Journal of Pediatrics, 139,* 189–196.

Wolf, G. (2008, April 21). Want to remember everything you'll ever learn? Surrender to this algorithm. *Wired.* Retrieved April 2012, from http://www.wired.com/medtech/health/magazine/16-05/ff_wozniak?currentPage=all

Wynn, K. (1992). Addition and subtraction by human infants. *Nature, 358,* 749–750.

Yurgelun-Todd, D. A., & Killgore, W. D. (2006). Fear-related activity in the prefrontal cortex increases with age during adolescence: A preliminary fMRI study. *Neuroscience Letters, 406,* 194–199.

INDEX